Mediating Health Information

Mediating Health Information

The Go-Betweens in a Changing Socio-Technical Landscape

Edited by

C. Nadine Wathen
The University of Western Ontario, Canada

Sally Wyatt
Royal Netherlands Academy of Arts and Sciences

Roma Harris
The University of Western Ontario, Canada

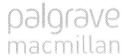

First published 2008 by
PALGRAVE MACMILLAN
Houndmills, Basingstoke, Hampshire RG21 6XS and
175 Fifth Avenue, New York, N.Y. 10010
Companies and representatives throughout the world

PALGRAVE MACMILLAN is the global academic imprint of the Palgrave Macmillan division of St. Martin's Press, LLC and of Palgrave Macmillan Ltd. Macmillan® is a registered trademark in the United States, United Kingdom and other countries. Palgrave is a registered trademark in the European Union and other countries.

ISBN-13: 978–0–230–20120–0   hardback
ISBN-10: 0–230–20120–2   hardback

This book is printed on paper suitable for recycling and made from fully managed and sustained forest sources. Logging, pulping and manufacturing processes are expected to conform to the environmental regulations of the country of origin.

A catalogue record for this book is available from the British Library.

Library of Congress Cataloging-in-Publication Data
Mediating health information : the go-between in a changing socio-technical landscape / [edited by] Nadine Wathen, Sally Wyatt, and Roma Harris.
    p. ; cm. — (Health, technology, and society)
Includes bibliographical references and indexes.
ISBN 0–230–20120–2 (alk. paper)
1. Communication in medicine. 2. Health education. 3. Medical informatics.
[DNLM: 1. Consumer Health Information—methods. 2. Consumer Health Information—trends. 3. Health Personnel. 4. Information Services—trends. 5. Information Systems—trends. 6. Librarians. WA 590 M48795 2008] I. Wathen, Nadine, 1968– II. Wyatt, Sally, 1959– III. Harris, Roma M. IV. Series.
R118.M417 2008
610.69'6—dc22   2008015927

10   9   8   7   6   5   4   3   2   1
17   16   15   14   13   12   11   10   09   08

Printed and bound in Great Britain by
CPI Antony Rowe, Chippenham and Eastbourne

Contents

List of Figures

Abbreviations and Acronyms

ACLU	American Civil Liberties Union
AHW	Aboriginal Health Worker
ALA	American Library Association
ALIA	Australian Library and Information Association
ALO	Aboriginal Liaison Officer
AOL	America Online
ASO	AIDS Service Organization
BCHG	British Columbia Health Guide
CHR	community health representative
CHW	community health worker
CIPA	Child Internet Protection Act (2002)
CIUS	Canadian Internet Use Survey
CLA	Canadian Library Association
CT	Computed Tomographic x-ray scan
CTC	community telehealth coordinator
DICOM	digital imaging and communications in medicine (standard format)
EBM	evidence-based-medicine
EEOC	Equal Employment Opportunity Commission
EHR	electronic health record
EMR	electronic medical record
FNIHB	First Nations Inuit Health Branch
HRT	hormone replacement therapy
ICTs	information and communication technologies
IM	instant messaging
ISP	internet server provider
KO	Keewaytinook Okimakanak Tribal Council
KOTH/M	Keewaytinook Okimakanak Telehealth/Telemedicine
M4M	men for men (websites)
MRI	Magnetic Resonance Imaging
MS	multiple sclerosis
MSN	Microsoft Network
NPH	'new public health'
OTN	Ontario Telemedicine Network

PACS	picture archive and communication systems
PHA	persons living with HIV/AIDS
PHR	personal health record
PICS	Platform for Internet Content Selection
STI	sexually transmitted infection
WAN	Wide Area Network

Acknowledgements

Many of the chapters in this book are the result of work supported in whole (Chapters 4 and 5) or in part (Chapters 1, 2, 3, 9, 10 and 11) by ACTION for Health, a four-year, $3 million project led by Ellen Balka at Simon Fraser University, Vancouver, Canada (http://www.sfu.ca/act4hlth/). The ACTION for Health project was supported by the Social Sciences and Humanities Research Council of Canada, through its Initiative for a New Economy Collaborative Research Initiative (grant number 512-2003-1017). One of the goals of ACTION for Health was to 'explore the use of the internet as a means of gaining access to health information, and specifically, to determine what roles information intermediaries (people and/or hardware and software who help information seekers find the information they need) fill when those around them seek health information via computers' (Balka, 2003). While exploring issues specific to computer-mediated health information-seeking, members of the project team, many of whom are contributors to this book, found that the concept of health information intermediation extended well beyond the use of specific technologies, or of technology in general. The exploration of convergences and divergences of theoretical ideas and empirical material generated from within and beyond the ACTION for Health project has resulted in the present volume. We are grateful to the ACTION for Health project for providing us with opportunities to meet and share our ideas. We would like to thank the contributors to this book, both those from ACTION for Health and those who came on board at a later stage, for their thoughtful contributions as well as for their responsiveness to our queries and proddings. We would also like to thank Andrew Webster, one of the editors of the *Health, Technology and Society* series, for his prompt and encouraging responses. The efforts of the staff at Palgrave Macmillan in seeing this book though to its present form are also greatly appreciated.

We thank the following for their permission to reproduce materials: Keewaytinook Okimakanak Tribal Council, Canada (Figure 8.1); Public Health Information Development Unit, University of Adelaide, Australia (Figure 9.1). We also thank Irene Gotz for creating Figures 1.1 and 1.2.

We are also grateful to The University of Western Ontario and the Royal Netherlands Academy of Arts and Sciences for their financial support of this project.

Series Editors' Preface

Medicine, health care, and the wider social meaning and management of health are undergoing major changes. In part this reflects developments in science and technology, which enable new forms of diagnosis, treatment and the delivery of health care. It also reflects changes in the locus of care and burden of responsibility for health. Today, genetics, informatics, imaging and integrative technologies, such as nanotechnology, are redefining our understanding of the body, health and disease; at the same time, health is no longer simply the domain of conventional medicine, nor the clinic.

More broadly, the social management of health itself is losing its anchorage in collective social relations and shared knowledge and practice, whether at the level of the local community or through state-funded socialised medicine. This individualisation of health is both culturally driven and state sponsored, as the promotion of 'self-care' demonstrates. The very technologies that redefine health are also the means through which this individualisation can occur – through 'e-health', diagnostic tests, and the commodification of restorative tissue, such as stem cells and cloned embryos.

This Series explores these processes *within* and *beyond* the conventional domain of 'the clinic', and asks whether they amount to a qualitative shift in the social ordering and value of medicine and health. Locating technical developments in wider socio-economic and political processes, each text discusses and critiques recent developments within health technologies in specific areas, drawing on a range of analyses provided by the social sciences. Some will have a more theoretical, others a more applied focus, interrogating and contributing towards a health policy. All will draw on recent research conducted by the author(s).

The Health, Technology and Society Series also looks toward the medium term in anticipating the likely configurations of health in advanced industrial societies and does so comparatively, through exploring the globalisation and the internationalisation of health, health inequalities and their expression through existing and new social divisions.

This book makes an important contribution to our understanding of the relationship between information and communication technologies

(ICTs) and health. Often this issue is explored solely through examining ICTs in the clinical domain. This book not only addresses this but is much broader in scope, to include the role of ICTs in non-clinical settings, such as libraries, minority communities, and the virtual world. What is especially valuable is that the editors have provided a strong conceptual framework used in each of the chapters, centred around the notion of the 'circuit of culture', and the inter-mediating role that ICTs may play here. The book also has a strong international focus that provides for a rich, comparative analysis and one that will appeal to many different academic and policy communities working across the ICT/health boundaries.

Andrew Webster and Sally Wyatt

Notes on the Editors and Contributors

The editors

Nadine Wathen is an assistant professor in the Faculty of Information & Media Studies at The University of Western Ontario, London, Ontario, Canada. She holds a Canadian Institutes of Health Research-Ontario Women's Health Council New Investigator Award to support her research, which examines women's health decision-making, including intervention research in the area of violence against women; projects to translate and mobilize research evidence in women's health to policy and practice, and projects on how people living in rural areas seek and use health information. Email: nwathen@uwo.ca.

Sally Wyatt is Professor of Digital Cultures in Development at Maastricht University and a senior research fellow with the Virtual Knowledge Studio for the Humanities and Social Sciences, Royal Netherlands Academy of Arts and Sciences. Her research focuses on the relationship between technological and social change, focusing particularly on issues of social exclusion and inequality. She has been president of the European Association for the Study of Science and Technology (2000–4) She has edited (with Flis Henwood, Nod Miller and Peter Senker) *Technology and In/equality: Questioning the Information Society* (Routledge, 2000). Email: sally.wyatt@vks.knaw.nl.

Roma Harris is a professor in the Faculty of Information and Media Studies at The University of Western Ontario. She has written about the impact of technological change on women's work in libraries and has been involved in a number of studies of help information-seeking by abused women. Currently, her work focuses on health help-seeking in rural communities and she is leading the 'Rural HIV/AIDS Information Networks Project' funded by the Canadian Institutes of Health Research. Harris is a founding member of two agencies to serve abused women as well as London's Centre for Education & Research on Violence Against Women and Children. Email: harris@uwo.ca.

The contributors

Ellen Balka is a professor in Simon Fraser University's School of Communication, where she also serves as director of the Assessment of Technology in Context Design Lab. She is Senior Research Scientist at Vancouver Coastal Health Research Institute's Centre for Clinical Epidemiology and Evaluation, and was recently awarded a Michael Smith Foundation for Health Research Senior Scholar award. Ellen's research focuses on issues related to the use of information technology for the production, consumption and use of health information. She is particularly interested in issues related to gender and inequality, and whether or not information technology contributes to or challenges gender and ethnic inequalities. She served as the principal investigator of the ACTION for Heath research programme, a four-year $3 million project funded by Canada's Social Sciences and Humanities Research Council of Canada, between 2003 and 2008. Email: ellenb@sfu.ca.

Leslie Bella is a research professor from Newfoundland's Memorial University, where she taught social work. She also held faculty positions at University of Alberta and University of Regina. Her social work practice and research focus on marginalized populations, and she has worked extensively with community centres in low-income communities, with the LGBTQ community, with aboriginal communities in Canada, and with a variety of community-based violence prevention initiatives. Her research has focused on caring labour, in a variety of community contexts, in formal health care and within the family. Email: lbella@tcc.on.ca.

Samantha Burdett is a professional librarian and researcher. She is also a part-time lecturer in the Faculty of Information & Media Studies at The University of Western Ontario. Email: sburdett@uwo.ca.

Arsalan Butt is a PhD student in Simon Fraser University's School of Communication and a data manager at the British Columbia Children's Hospital. His research focuses on socio-political aspects of technology, with a particular interest in issues related to the political use of ICTs; intellectual property protection (particularly in developing countries); and health technology. He has published in the fields of medicine, health technology and technoethics. Email: ab@sfu.ca.

Debbie Chaves obtained her doctorate in biophysics from the University of Guelph in 1999. While raising her pre-school children, she taught first-year physics at various Ontario universities. Earning a Master of

Library and Information Science from The University of Western Ontario in 2007, she is now science librarian at Wilfrid Laurier University. Her research is eclectic, working with information-seeking activities of physicists, history of the science, technology and medicine books of the Pioneer Collection and issues relating to consumer health. Email: dchaves@uoguelph.ca.

Jana Fear is a planner with the South West Local Health Integration Network, London, Ontario, Canada. She has worked as a research assistant in the Faculty of Information and Media Studies at The University of Western Ontario. Her research involves understanding how people seek and use health information and the role of technologies (particularly the internet) in the communication of that information. Email: jana.fear@sympatico.ca.

Adam Fiser is a PhD candidate in the Faculty of Information Studies and a graduate fellow of the Knowledge Media Design Institute at the University of Toronto. He is a researcher with the Canadian Research Alliance on Community Innovation and Networking and the Community Wireless Infrastructure Research Project. His research focuses on the political, economic and organizational aspects of emerging broadband technologies, particularly in the context of remote indigenous community networks. Email: adam.fiser@gmail.com.

Elaine Gibson is Associate Professor of Law and Associate Director of the Health Law Institute at Dalhousie Law Faculty, Halifax, Nova Scotia, Canada. Her areas of expertise include health law, privacy law and liability for negligence. Elaine participates in a number of research projects concerning electronic health information, focusing on the uses of information in the areas of health research and public health surveillance. She is co-editor (with Jocelyn Downie) of *Health Law at the Supreme Court of Canada* (Irwin Law, 2007). Elaine was recipient of the Virtual Scholar in Residence Award (2005–6) co-sponsored by the Law Commission of Canada and the Social Sciences and Humanities Research Council. Email: Elaine.Gibson@dal.ca.

Penny Gill is a graduate of Memorial University of Newfoundland's Master's of Social Work programme. Originally from Prince Edward Island, she received her BSW from St Thomas University in Fredericton. She practices Social Work in Truro, Nova Scotia with the Mental Health Family First Community Outreach programme and works as a men's counsellor at Bridges, a domestic abuse counseling centre. She is hoping to expand her knowledge of narrative therapy, particularly with aggressive teens and teens who abuse their parents. Email: gill_penny2003@yahoo.ca.

Michelle Hall is a researcher in the Service Leadership and Innovation Research Program at Queensland University of Technology, Australia. Michelle is currently completing her Master of Business (Research) at QUT, exploring the relationship between consumption practices and place-based communities, and the ways in which servicescapes can help to build social networks. Email: ml.hall@qut.edu.au.

Flis Henwood is Professor of Social Informatics in the School of Computing, Mathematical and Information Sciences at the University of Brighton, where she heads the Social Informatics Research Unit (www.brighton.ac.uk/cmis/research/groups/siru). Her most recent work focuses on the implementation and use of information and communication technologies in health care. She has published widely on e-health issues in both academic journals and peer-reviewed professional/ practitioner journals. She co-edited (with Ellen Balka) an 'e-Health' special issue of the journal *Information, Communication and Society* in 2005. Her publications have appeared in a range of disciplinary fields, including sociology of medicine, social policy, information systems and media studies. Email: f.henwood@bton.ac.uk.

Judith Krajnak is an independent evaluation consultant. For the last three years, she has also taught a program evaluation course designed for health practitioners working in regional health settings. Her applied interests include evaluating e-health programmes targeting how the public obtains and uses web-based health information. Email: jkrajnak@earthlink.net.

Susan Leggett is a researcher in the Service Leadership and Innovation Research Programme at the Queensland University of Technology, Australia. She has taken part in a series of research projects in rural and remote communities in Queensland, focusing on technological support for geographically isolated rural women, for mental health and suicide prevention workers, and for health intermediaries. Email: s.leggett@qut.edu.au.

Robert Luke is Director, Applied Research and Innovation for George Brown College in Toronto, Ontario, Canada, and a researcher at the University of Toronto's Knowledge Media Design Institute. His research interests involve Community Learning Networks, with a particular emphasis on learning environments for health and education. This includes work on online inter-professional education for health care teams, as well as for patient learning. His research agenda is guided by active involvement in the development of standards and technologies that assist people with various abilities and learning styles. This is explored through community informatics and the design of information systems that enhance community social, economic, and political development. Email: rluke@georgebrown.ca.

Audrey Marshall is a senior lecturer in the School of Computing, Mathematical and Information Sciences at the University of Brighton and a Senior Research Fellow with the Social Informatics Research Unit. She has worked in a range of library and information sectors, including public libraries and health information services, and is an active member of CILIP, the professional body for library and information specialists in the UK. Her research interests revolve around the uses of information and information and communication technologies in a health context, focusing particularly on issues of partnership and participation. Email: a.m.marshall@brighton.ac.uk.

Peter S. Pennefather is a professor in the Leslie Dan Faculty of Pharmacy, University of Toronto. He is co-founder and academic director of the Laboratory for Collaborative Diagnostics. His current research focuses on new approaches for imaging and monitoring cell function using commodity consumer electronics technology with the goal of defining new and sustainable ways of acquiring digital diagnostic and analytical information needed in coordinating health care. He is involved in a number of education and research initiatives concerning inter-professional collaboration and dialogue. Email: p.pennefather@utoronto.ca.

Irving Rootman is Chair of the Health and Learning Knowledge Centre at the University of Victoria and Co-chair of the Canadian Public Health Association Expert Panel on Health Literacy. He has published widely in the area of health promotion and served as Technical Advisor, Consultant and Senior Scientist for the World Health Organization. He has also been a member of the Health Promotion and Disease Prevention Advisory Board and the Health Literacy Committee of the US Institute of Medicine, as well as the Board of the International Union for Health Promotion and Education. Email: irootman@uvic.ca.

T. C. Sanders is a doctoral candidate in the Department of Sociology at York University, Toronto, Ontario, Canada. His primary research interest concerns public access to and use of digital technology, commonly referred to as the 'digital divide'. His other areas of research include the sociology of health and illness, HIV/AIDS and the use of the internet as a methodological research tool. Email: tcs@yorku.ca.

Lyn Simpson is Assistant Dean in the Faculty of Business and researcher in the Service Leadership and Innovation Research Programme at the Queensland University of Technology, Brisbane, Australia. Lyn has conducted extensive research projects funded by the Australian Research Council in the areas of social and policy implications of communication technologies for sustainable development in rural communities. Lyn is particularly interested in the impacts of communication technology on community social capital, capacity-building and rural community development. Her most recent projects have focused on the ways ICTs can support health literacy and health outcomes particularly in remote and indigenous communities. Email: le.simpson@qut.edu.au.

West Suhanic is co-founder and academic director of the Laboratory for Collaborative Diagnostics at the University of Toronto, Canada. His current research is focused on digital, distributed diagnostic devices to collect and populate meta-data rich image formats such as BIOTIFF. In addition he is investigating the use of instant messaging and onion routing technology as new infrastructure technologies to give health imaging more accessible agency while protecting individuals' privacy. Email: west.suhanic@gmail.com.

Jan Sutherland is a research associate at the Health Law Institute, Dalhousie University, Halifax, Nova Scotia. She has an MA (Philosophy) and an LLB. With Elaine Gibson, she is currently researching legal issues relating to the application of information technologies in health care. She has particular interest in issues in public health. Email: jsuther3@dal.ca.

Tiffany Veinot is a PhD candidate at the Faculty of Information and Media Studies at the University of Western Ontario. Her doctoral research focuses on exchange of HIV/AIDS information through social networks in rural Canadian communities. Her research interests include understanding health information exchange within communities; investigating health information service models for marginalized populations; and using sociological theories of knowledge to study the socio-cultural production of information. Email: tveinot@uwo.ca.

1
The Go-Betweens: Health, Technology and Info(r)mediation

Sally Wyatt, Roma Harris and Nadine Wathen

Welcome or not, most people in Western countries are unable to get through a day without receiving a dose of health information. It is available from, passed through or pushed at health help seekers by health care professionals, alternative health care practitioners, pharmaceutical companies, employers, co-workers, friends, family members, vendors of health products and through government-sponsored health promotion campaigns. It is delivered through a variety of media, including self-help books, magazines, leaflets, television and radio advertising and programming and, increasingly, the internet. If the volume of health information present in the public domain in previous decades could be described as a mountain, the current situation might better be described as an avalanche. Recipes or directives about practices for healthy living, as well as information about medical conditions and treatments, prescription drugs and alternative health products and therapies, are everywhere. Against this dense backdrop of advice is the increasingly prevalent notion in public health policy that people, whether as patients, care providers, citizens or, increasingly, consumers, have an obligation to keep themselves informed about health matters.

How are ordinary people taking up the challenge to locate, retrieve, receive, digest and cope with the mass of health information available? What are the roles of technologies and human helpers that mediate between health information sources and health 'consumers' or end-users? In this book we explore the largely unexplored 'middle' space of human and technical mediators in the health information process. To investigate this sometimes mysterious middle, we have brought together contributions from research undertaken in different countries (Canada, Australia, United Kingdom) in which various aspects of the health information exchange process are explored.

To illustrate the complexities of health information exchange we introduce a brief, fictional example.[1]

> Ms. Smith has been taking hormone replacement therapy (HRT) for five years and it has made her feel much better, relieving the most acute symptoms of menopause. A friend recently gave her a copy of a popular women's magazine, which carried an article about different treatments for menopausal symptoms. The article discussed some of the risks associated with HRT, including an increased chance of breast cancer. Ms. Smith visits her family doctor, Dr. Jones, for her regular check-up and a repeat prescription, but she also wants to know what he thinks about the long-term risks of HRT. While at the doctor's office, the nurse performs a breast examination and gives Ms. Smith some leaflets about mammograms. Ms. Smith is especially concerned as her sister was recently diagnosed with breast cancer and she has been spending a lot of time with her recently.
>
> There are several types of mediation going on here: between Ms. Smith and her friend, between Ms. Smith and her sister, between Ms. Smith and Dr. Jones and the nurse, and between Ms. Smith and the leaflets and the magazine article. The leaflets were prepared by the health authority and designed to be used across the country. The article was written by a journalist, living hundreds of kilometres away. The article conforms to the magazine's editorial policy about how to report research results, a policy which is different from that of the *Journal of the American Medical Association*, which Ms. Smith does not read.
>
> The situation quickly becomes more complex when Ms. Smith watches a TV chat show during which a famous older actress talks about how HRT has changed her life. Ms. Smith goes online to look at some of the websites mentioned in the magazine article, in the leaflets the nurse gave her and at the end of the chat show. From these, she starts clicking and linking. When she tries to do this again with a friend at her local library, she cannot find some of the information she found when using her own PC. The local library has installed filtering software on its public access computers to prevent children from accessing pornography and sex education information, but neither Ms. Smith nor some of the library staff are aware of this or its impact on access to health sites.

In this example we see how technologies – in this case, television, the internet and computer software – as well as places – the home, the library and the doctor's office – can play a role in mediating health information.

Mediation: pipelines, transforming conduits or Chinese whispers?

In this book we follow Latour (2005) in distinguishing between an intermediary and a mediator. He explains the distinction as follows:

> An *intermediary*, in my vocabulary, is what transports meaning or force without transformation: defining its inputs is enough to define its outputs. For all practical purposes, an intermediary can be taken not only as a black box, but also as a black box counting for one, even if it is internally made of many parts. *Mediators*, on the other hand, cannot be counted as just one; they might count for one, for nothing, for several, or for infinity. Their input is never a good predictor of their output; their specificity has to be taken into account every time. Mediators transform, translate, distort, and modify the meaning of the elements they are supposed to carry. No matter how *complicated* an intermediary is, it may, for all practical purposes, count for just one – or even for nothing at all because it can be easily forgotten. No matter how apparently simple a mediator may look, it may become *complex*; it may lead in multiple directions which will modify all the contradictory accounts attributed to its role. A properly functioning computer could be taken as a good case of a complicated intermediary while a banal conversation may become a terribly complex chain of mediators where passions, opinions, and attitudes bifurcate at every turn. But if it breaks down, a computer may turn into a horrendously complex mediator while a highly sophisticated panel during an academic conference may become a perfectly predictable and uneventful intermediary in rubber stamping a decision made elsewhere.
>
> (Latour, 2005: 39; emphasis in original)

We are primarily interested in mediators and mediation because, as the chapters in this book demonstrate, health information is rarely, if ever, intermediated in a simple, straightforward way. The fantasy of some policy-makers, played on by technology vendors, is that information can be sent easily from its source to its intended recipients, and that it will not be affected by the medium or by the context in which the recipients are situated, including factors such as their health situation, living arrangements and education. This is what Latour means by intermediation. Figure 1.1 illustrates this ideal as a simple download from machine to brain. In this book, we explore the much more interesting, and real, situations in which information is produced, distributed, regulated and

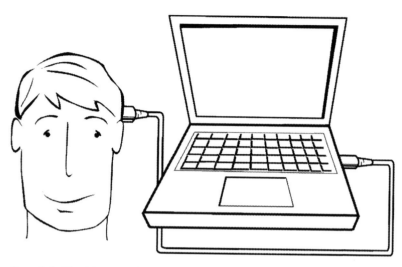

Figure 1.1   The 'clean pipeline': an idealized view of information intermediaries

used. 'Health information' in its broadest sense is itself produced within local contexts by individuals and groups with a wide range of interests, such as scientists in research laboratories, health professionals in clinical settings, manufacturers of health and beauty products, peer support groups such as Alzheimer's societies, organic produce growers or African politicians who claim that AIDS is a curable disease. The information produced by these different sources is transformed by others, ranging from professionals attached to the formal medical system (doctors, nurses, librarians, pharmacists) to those outside the system (health food store operators or shamanic elders in Aboriginal communities). As health help seekers, ordinary people, whether they are 'health-concerned' patients or providing care for others, attempt to make sense of this myriad of information in ways that will help them in their particular and local circumstances. This is illustrated in Figure 1.2, which shows the myriad information sources that people make sense of and navigate all the time.

The people who mediate are situated between the information sources and the information seekers. They effect the transfer of information that can be derived from a variety of sources, through a variety of means, to others who are seeking information or who might be expected to seek such information in the future. In addition to all the traditional mediators, with the widespread diffusion of ICTs, new mediators are emerging, including software designers, website producers, makers of digital images and others. On occasion, the technologies themselves, whether software

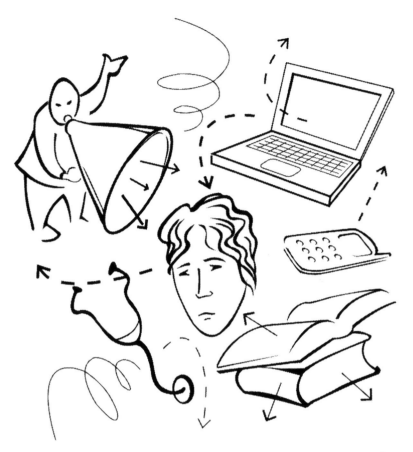

Figure 1.2 The messy reality: 'info(r)mediation' as experienced by health information seekers

filters (Gibson and Sutherland, this volume), avatars (Sanders, this volume), diagnostic digital images (Pennefather and Suhanic, this volume) or government-sponsored health portals (Balka and Butt, this volume) can appear to have agency as mediators in their own right.

We use the term health 'info(r)mediator' to refer to people, as well as various configurations of people and technologies, that perform the mediating work involved in enabling health information seekers to locate, retrieve, understand, cope with and use the information for which they are looking. This is consistent with Latour's use of mediation, as we share his emphasis on and interest in the transforming and distorting (Harris et al., this volume) power of mediators. His use of mediator is quite general, and by adding 'info' we signal our focus on the mediation of (health) information. For us, infomediation refers to the inevitable, if not always predictable, transformation that occurs as information is conveyed from one place, person or situation to another. Info(r)mediation, however, is used to draw attention to those situations in which the human mediators convey information in order to effect change in the behaviour or actions of those looking for information. For example, Bella et al. (this volume) distinguish between those health care professions that aim to provide people with information, but which leave subsequent action to the discretion of the people involved, and other professions that aim to change behaviour through the provision of information. Thus, the '(r)' draws attention to the way in which compliance or coercion is sometimes implied in the info(r)mediating process.

The concept of info(r)mediation, as it is explored in this book, has received relatively little attention in the health or social sciences. In the health sciences, the scant existing literature focuses primarily on intermediation of data between large, complex information management systems and individuals, usually administrators. Similarly, one can find mention of data/information intermediation by intelligent software agents and the like in the computing science and human–computer interaction literatures. The idea in both conceptualizations of information intermediation is that the volume and complexity of health-related data collected by health systems require approaches, preferably automated ones, to mine, filter and report selected data to those who may require it. The types of decisions represented as requiring informational support in these studies are generally administrative (in the form of cost-cutting, error-reducing and/or general quality control or improvement decisions) (O'Kane, 2002; de Brantes et al., 2007), or in some cases geared towards more commercial applications (Hagel and Rayport, 1997).

In a treatment of the topic by Song and Zehadi (2007), insights from e-commerce and actor-network theory are combined to analyse users' trust in health infomediaries. For Song and Zahedi, infomediaries provide 'unbiased information about a variety of medical, health and wellness topics for [users'] health-related decision-making as well as information about various health providers' (2007: 391). Their reliance on the notion of 'unbiased information' makes their concept of infomediary closer to Latour's definition of intermediary, whereas we use it to draw attention to the mediation, transformation, translation and sometimes distortion of information. And, as we will see in some of the chapters in this book, notably those by Bella et al. and Harris et al., the degree of 'bias' and the intent of health mediation vary depending on the positioning of the information 'giver' and the 'receiver' in the exchange process.

The contributors to this book are interested in the ways in which humans and non-humans mediate, either together or at a distance from one another, the huge volume of uncertain and sometimes contradictory health information. While practitioners such as physicians, nurses, pharmacists, social workers and librarians may assume health mediating roles as part of their jobs, to what extent are they professionally prepared to do so? For instance, even though librarians may be skilled in identifying users' needs and linking information seekers to reliable sources, they may have little formal training in the area of health and may therefore have legitimate ethical and legal concerns about providing what might be regarded as 'medical' advice (Henwood et al., this volume). Alternatively, although health professionals are ethically bound to provide the best possible care for their patients, they may have little formal preparation as patient 'educators' and limited skills in information retrieval or 'shared decision-making'. Regardless of such limitations, however, health care providers are increasingly expected to perform these roles, especially in response to '(mis)informed' patients who arrive for health care visits with information they have found on their own, often on the internet. In this book we also consider mediation as it is performed by those who have no formal link to the health care system, for example, lay people who pass on health information to others in their social networks. Should we think of their roles as 'info(r)meddling' or do they positively facilitate the health information seeking process?

The role of lay people or 'informal' mediators has already received attention in the literature about users and technology. Friends, family members, neighbours and colleagues often serve as key links between people, technology and health information. Bakardjieva (2005) introduced the notion of the 'warm expert' – someone with technical competence who is in a position to help a new internet user. A warm expert mediates between the specialized knowledge and skills necessary to use the technology and the specific situation and needs of the 'novice' with whom the 'expert' has some kind of personal relationship. Bakardjieva finds that warm experts are essential in assisting in the process of learning and appropriation, even when novice users have followed formal courses of instruction. Of course, this is not confined to ICTs, nor is it a completely new concept. For example, many people draw on the goodwill and competence of their friends, neighbours and relatives when learning to drive a car or install a DVD. Further, the value of informal learning has been shown to be important for helping inexperienced users become familiar with machines. Most importantly, for our purposes here, help with equipment and software is not enough at the individual or social level to enable people to make sense of the complex information they may find when seeking to inform themselves about health issues. Warm experts can be crucial for helping people to incorporate computers and the internet into their everyday practices, but Wyatt et al. (2005) have extended the notion to include helping people understand the relevance of health information for their own situations. Particularly in the case of complex medical literature, many people are at an understandable loss to know what it means for their own situation. For example, when applying the results of clinical research to the treatment of individual patients, even physicians face a significant challenge in translating the information because of the 'inherent uncertainty' of such evidence (Griffiths et al., 2005: 1). Stewart (2007) uses the term 'local expert' to highlight the ways in which expertise is relative and only made salient within local contexts of the home, workplaces, groups of friends, and so on. This perspective enables him to demonstrate how individuals (whom we would described as locally situated info(r)mediators) can act as bridges, transferring their knowledge across different local contexts. Stewart also draws attention to the possibility that this role can put a strain on relationships by introducing divisions of labour or power/knowledge differences that are not always easy to manage within personal relationships. A further necessary qualification, raised by Harris et al., is that warm experts do not necessarily provide helpful or accurate information.

Studies of help and information seeking have repeatedly identified a set of common characteristics that are shared by people who have been identified as most helpful by those seeking assistance (Harris and Dewdney, 1994). The actual role of effective help and information providers in relation to the help seeker, whether they are professional experts, police officers, community service workers, volunteers, family members, neighbours or friends, often seems to be almost incidental to whether the support they provide is perceived to be valuable by those receiving help. People who are praised for their helpfulness are generally described as warm, supportive, concerned and non-judgemental, and they are appreciated for taking the time necessary to listen carefully and respectfully to others' inquiries and concerns. These communication behaviours comprise the foundation of the facilitative relationship that is a significant element of 'doing' effective information exchange.

Having discussed some of the potential roles of human mediators, we briefly turn to mediation at a distance, still involving people but incorporating more complex socio-technical configurations. The extension of such configurations across time and space is largely the result of developments in ICTs, from the printing press to radio, television and now including networked computers. An important consideration throughout this book is the effect of the medium on the process of health information exchange, and we focus on information and communication technologies (ICTs), their various configurations and their effects on the process of health info(r)mediation. Further questions include: To what extent do ICTs enable access to information that would otherwise not be accessible and do they present particular contextual circumstances that may help or hinder not only access, but also comprehension and utility? How are ICTs used by professional and informal mediators on behalf of others who are seeking health information, and what additional complexity do they bring to the information-seeking process? What are the different human–machine configurations that help people or hinder them from making sense of an ever-increasing volume of health information? Does the increased availability of computer-mediated information disrupt relationships between those needing information and those providing it, and if so, how? What is the influence of norms and standards that guide the production and distribution of health information and which may be more or less visible to patients and human mediators?

Thompson (1995) draws attention to differences between face-to-face interaction, mediated interaction (letter writing, telephone) and mediated quasi-interaction (mass media). He highlights the dialogical nature of the first two and the greater range of symbolic resources available in face-to-face interaction. While this can be useful for analysing changes in the time–space dimensions of different media,[2] Thompson does idealize face-to-face interaction for its richness and clarity. In Latour's terms, face-to-face interaction is, for Thompson, a form of intermediation. In this book, we do not privilege face-to-face interaction in that way. The results of the research presented in later chapters demonstrate repeatedly that even if personal health experiences are being communicated face-to-face, they are also being mediated, in Latour's sense of the information being transformed, translated or even distorted. Similarly, we do not valorize the 'self-service' imperative implicitly or explicitly advocated by those promoting the broad adoption of e-health systems that encourage citizens to behave as consumers of health information supported by technologies (such as the government health web portals described by Balka and Butt, this volume).

Health info(r)mediation is not a simple exchange between a patient and some information, or between a patient and another person. There are many social actors and systems of rules and technologies that may be involved in health information exchange, including patients, members of their social networks, medical professionals and the rules governing their conduct, information professionals with their own codes of practice, health educators, journalists, publishers, copyright lawyers, computer, network/internet and software providers, as well as local and national governments. In the next section, we present the framework that we have adopted in this book for making sense of the different actors and processes involved in the production, distribution and consumption of information.

Coping with complexity: The circuit of culture

We have chosen Stuart Hall's 'circuit of culture' (1997; du Gay et al., 1997) to make sense of the complexity (different from 'complicated' – see the Latour quote above) of mediators and mediation processes. We do this in order to situate the actors and rules, and to analyse all the possible places and processes that might affect the ways in which people make, exchange, find and use health information. The 'circuit' comprises the processes of representation, identity, production, consumption and regulation which together provide a framework for analysis (see Figure 1.3). This framework is useful for understanding how health information is represented, what social identities are associated with it, how it is

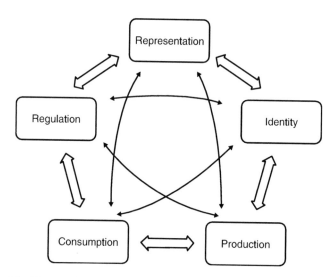

Figure 1.3 Circuit of culture (adapted from du Gay et al., 1997: 3)

produced and consumed, and what legal frameworks and ethical norms regulate its distribution and use. It enables us to analyse all the possible places and processes that might affect the ways in which people make, exchange, find and use health information.

Each of the chapters deploys one or more of the five processes in order to address the following sorts of analytical questions:

- *Consumption*: How do people obtain and use or absorb health information? What channels and media are involved? Does the medium matter?
- *Production*: How is health information produced? By whom and for what purposes? Does the medium make a difference to the ways in which information is structured and accessed?
- *Regulation*: What mechanisms regulate the distribution and use of the information? What copyright rules are in place? What mechanisms regulate the role(s) of the mediator (human, technical or both) and/or the (intended and perhaps unintended) users of the information?
- *Identity*: What social identities are associated with the production and consumption of health information? Who is the intended audience? Are these identities changing as the available technologies for distributing information change?
- *Representation*: How are health information, patients and health-mediating relationships represented in various contexts, such as policy documents, health education materials and newspapers? Representation through language is central to the processes by which meaning is produced. Meaning can be produced at multiple locations and can then circulate through different processes or practices.

There are also interactions between the processes. For example, the ways in which information is produced structure and limit how and by whom it can be consumed; the intellectual property regime influences what information is produced; the identities of professional groups are important for understanding the ways in which information is produced and distributed; and the representation of social groups in policy documents affects the ways that the social group not only sees itself, but also how it consumes health information.

Patelis (2000) attempts something similar in her analysis of America Online. She introduces the concept of 'e-mediation' to draw attention to the ways in which telecommunication, software, service providers, navigation tools and content interact to structure the content available to users. She is particularly concerned to demonstrate how the content available to individual users is not neutral, but is structured by the interests of hardware, software and content providers. Although her approach takes into account how production, regulation and representation structure user experiences, it leaves very little space for the agency of users, captured by the processes of consumption and identity. Thus, we prefer the circuit of culture, as it enables us to consider both structure and agency. In particular, the chapters by Fiser and Luke and by Simpson et al. about the use of ICTs in remote regions of Canada and Australia, respectively, analyse the interplay between long-standing structures of social and health inequalities and the agency of Indigenous peoples.

The separation of the five processes in the 'circuit of culture' is an analytic device, and it is important to remember this is a 'circuit'. Thus, it does not matter where one starts and, in reality, the five processes are intertwined. These two analytic devices, namely the circuit of culture and info(r)mediation, enable us – the editors and contributors to this book – to structure our analyses of the processes by which health information is mediated and to take account of the multiplicity and complexity of mediation processes. They have other advantages: neither privileges one type of actor or process over any other; many different human–medium–information configurations can be considered; we can be symmetrical in focusing on things that work as well as those that do not, as well as in our treatment of visible and invisible work and technologies, and formal and informal work.

Organization of the book

This book focuses on what ICTs mean for both professional and lay understandings of health information, as well as communication about health matters. These are important considerations in terms of the shifting loci of health diagnoses and treatment, as well as responsibility for health. Beck (1992) argues that processes of individualization are furthered by the risk society as individuals are thrown back on themselves. This book contributes to debates about the risk society in that it brings to the fore the ways in which ICTs make available enormous amounts of information about risks which individuals have to negotiate and make sense of for themselves. However, rather than seeing this simply or even primarily as a process of individualization, this book focuses on the ways in which ICTs reconfigure social relationships and responsibilities. Contributions to the book are concerned with a variety of applications of ICTs to the mediation of health information, including digitized imaging, software filters, avatars and web portals. However, the focus is on the everyday and situated practices of use. The authors of the chapters go well beyond the conventional domain of the 'clinic' as a privileged site of health information exchange by drawing on empirical work that considers sites such as libraries and on- and off-line communities, including remote communities of Indigenous peoples.

The book is not formally divided into parts or sections; however, there is a logic guiding the chapter order. In Chapter 2, Bella et al. explore how the health information exchange function is conceived of and practised in different professions through an analysis of course materials and codes of practice, and how technology is embedded in this function. Six occupations are analysed in which health info(r)mediation is a significant aspect of practice, including general practice medicine, nursing, social work (particularly in health settings), dietetics and nutrition, pharmacy and librarianship. The ways in which info(r)mediation features in the professional identities of these occupations, how each group claims ground or 'turf' in relation to this function, how clients/patients/users/customers are positioned in relation to practitioners, what expectations exist with respect to the production of health information by practitioners for their clients, and how technology is incorporated into the performance of info(r)mediation work in each occupation are all examined.

Chapters 3 and 4 develop the library theme in different ways. Public libraries have long been important sites for health information access and support, and their role in this regard is increasingly being stressed by national and local government policies. As public libraries are also important sites of free internet access, it is envisaged that they may be expected to play a larger role as intermediaries in the health information-seeking practices of members of their local communities. How prepared are public libraries to perform this role? What are the expectations of library users in this regard? Henwood et al. address these questions by examining the ways in which library staff deal with health information enquiries in the context of increased availability of computers within public libraries and a growing emphasis on 'e-health'. Much existing literature on consumer health information seeking is framed, implicitly at least, within the 'e-health' discourse, which understands health information as empowering and the internet as a tool for accessing that information. In this discourse, public libraries are positioned as potential sites of health info(r)mediation, offering both specialist knowledge in information retrieval as well as free access to the internet to consumer-citizens who are active information seekers. Through an exploration of the practices involved in supporting health information seeking in the public library context, this chapter analyses how understanding e-health discourse can help make sense of the specific socio-technical configuration set up in the public library to support these practices and the challenges of delivering on the promise implied by these arrangements.

Technology is the focus in Gibson and Sutherland's chapter about the use of filtering software in public libraries, ostensibly to protect children from pornography but at the same time blocking many health information sites. Filters are designed to control the type of information that can be retrieved by computer users. As such, they are a technology that acts as an information mediator because they affect the ability of users to acquire information. Insofar as libraries apply filtering technology, library administrators are also implicated in the process of mediation, as their actions result in a transformation or biasing of the information available to information seekers. This chapter examines the use of content control filters meant to screen out inappropriate websites in the public library environment, as these institutions have been the focus of efforts to control access to information. The prevalence of health information on the internet is described, as is the nature of filters and their effect on searches for health information. The legal regimes of four countries – Canada, the United States, the United Kingdom and Australia – are surveyed with respect to internet censorship and filters. The ways in which public libraries have responded to the pressures to install filters are the main focus of the chapter, which concludes with a brief discussion of the ethical issues raised by this type of technology.

The importance of technological forms of mediation, of which filters are an example, is also pursued in Chapters 5, 6 and 7. Balka and Butt examine the software underlying a government-sponsored online health information service. This chapter draws attention to the ways that hardware and software configurations function as information mediators, in two ways. First, as with the previous chapter, Balka and Butt analyse how the software itself is black-boxed, making it very difficult for users to know how search engines work. They also demonstrate how different configurations render some kinds of information visible (how long people waited in an emergency room before being seen), while rendering other kinds of information invisible (how sick those patients were who had to wait a long time in an emergency room). It is based on a study of the accessibility of a health website in search engines. The chapter focuses on the means through which software and hardware play a role in structuring the flow of information received by health information seekers, be they hospital administrators or teenaged web surfers looking for birth control information.

Pennefather and Suhanic focus on the role of digital diagnostic images used to document the causes of people's diseases and their state of health. These can range from digital x-rays (e.g. medical diagnostic imaging) to digital micrographs of a clinical sample (e.g. tissue-based diagnostics). Because diagnostic image files can now be easily embedded in electronic health records, which in turn could be increasingly accessible to patients themselves, there is now the potential to create a medium of communication between patients and their care providers who also have access to the electronic health record. Diagnostic images are highly constructed and interpreted artefacts that serve to 'etch' concepts about the physical body with political hierarchies and technical practices. Pennefather and Suhanic argue that patients' voices should be added to this construction by enabling them to communicate their desires and expectations about treatment and care, as information to be contained in the digital suitcase, alongside the images of their own bodies.

Sanders analyses a range of strategies that have been used to provide safe-sex information on men-for-men (M4M) websites. Since the late 1990s such websites and chat rooms have become increasingly popular among gay and bisexual men seeking casual sex partners. The websites are public, localized and offer free basic memberships, containing user-friendly search engines for locating other members, and boast thousands of members within most metropolitan areas. In recent years, these websites have been implicated in outbreaks of sexually transmitted infections (STIs). Not surprisingly, researchers concerned with the health of gay and bisexual men have developed a keen interest in these websites as a potential source for studying risky sexual behaviour among men seeking men, as well as their potential for providing safe-sex and other sexual health information. The websites can function as vital health intermediaries between public health professionals and, broadly speaking, a population at high risk for STIs. A series of online health information strategies has been produced for public use on many M4M websites. The strategies range from passive online notifications and health advisory links to interactive websites and chat room-based educators. These interventions are produced with unidirectional intent, namely to disseminate specific information that, ideally, influences or modifies the sexual behaviour of the M4M community, to gain 'compliance' as Bella et al. discuss in their chapter. Seen in this light, however, the relationship between ICTs and people appears purely deterministic and fixed, instead of negotiated and fluid. This chapter analyses such online health strategies as mediator or contested medium, in play between the health community and M4M website users.

In Chapters 8, 9 and 10, the focus shifts to the range of human–technology configurations for providing health information and support in Indigenous and rural/remote communities in Canada and Australia. Technology promises to deliver health information to sparsely populated communities that can take days to reach by land (or even longer during the Canadian winter). Fiser and Luke provide a nuanced analysis of the role of information intermediaries in First Nations (Indigenous) communities in northwestern Ontario, neither rejecting nor celebrating the promise of technology. Since 1998, a coalition of First Nations in this remote region has sought to overcome their geographic constraints and augment district health care services with computer-mediated communications using a community-based network. The initial objective was to design a web-supported health communication system that could address some of the health needs of First Nations in the remote Sioux Lookout Zone. The system was designed, in its initial conception, to support delivery of health care at a distance by allowing medical specialists based in urban centres to interact with patients and their local health care providers using web-supported videoconferencing and related technologies. This chapter describes the evolution of this telemedicine system to a more broadly used and useful community health tool, focusing not only on the apparent mismatches between the system and the existing culture of use in the communities (mismatches that result in the potential usefulness of the system not been fully exploited) but, of interest to our discussion, the emergence of a new info(r)mediator role – the community telehealth coordinator.

Simpson et al. investigate how Aboriginal health workers engage with the role of health information intermediary in Indigenous communities in Australia. The discussion focuses on how this role is represented in government policy and identified in practice by the communities and the health workers themselves, especially with respect to the extent of use and usefulness of technology for these essential links in the health provision chain. The divergence between policy representation and practical identification as played out through regulation is explored, specifically in the ways that Aboriginal health workers are resourced and supported by their employers and the communities they serve. Both Simpson et al. and Fiser and Luke highlight tensions between the focus on the individual within Western medicine and the more community-oriented notions of well-being within Indigenous communities, and explore the unpredictable ways in which ICTs are developed and used in such settings.

Harris et al. remain in rural (often remote) areas in Canada and pick up the very important notion of misinformation, and how it may be transmitted. The informal exchange of health-related information is an important support process, particularly for people with limited access to formal health care services and professional providers. For people living with HIV/AIDS, geography can pose a special challenge because of the complexities of the disease and requirements to travel considerable distances for specialist care. Because HIV/AIDS is a disease that evokes fear, and because of flawed assumptions about its transmission and local epidemiology, information about HIV/AIDS may travel 'underground' in rural communities. HIV/AIDS can also inspire the exchange of information of dubious quality, such as medically unsubstantiated rumours about 'cures' or treatments, and conspiracy theories about its purported creation by governments or drug companies. In this chapter, the notion of 'misinfo(r)mediation' is explored, namely the exchange of misinformation about HIV/AIDS in rural settings in Canada, the impact on community members of sharing false or questionable information about the disease, and how people living with HIV/AIDS, their friends and family members, as well as health care and service providers 'mediate' or intervene to correct misunderstandings about HIV/AIDS.

In the final chapter, we draw conclusions and implications for health care and information-providing policy and practice. As the provision of health information is increasingly seen by governments as an alternative to the provision of health care itself, and as debates about self-care and individual responsibility gain attention, the policy implications of this book are of crucial importance.

Notes

1. While this story is fictional, it is based on work we have done about the ways in which women inform themselves about the symptoms and treatments of menopause, especially HRT (Henwood et al., 2003; Wathen, 2006a, 2006b; Wyatt and Henwood, 2006).
2. Thompson's distinctions are reminiscent of Innis' (1950, 1951) pioneering work on media, communication and power, in which he distinguishes between time-biased and space-biased media.

2

'Everybody's Talking at Me':[1] Situating the Client in the Info(r)mediary Work of the Health Professions

Leslie Bella, Roma Harris, Debbie Chavez, Jana Fear and Penny Gill

The widespread availability of health information via the internet has changed the nature of the health information exchange. Nettleton and Burrows argue that 'medical knowledge has *escaped* and is thus no longer something that can be accessed and, more importantly perhaps, produced and regulated by medical experts' (2003: 178). Within this changing environment, how do workers in the health professions position themselves and their patients or clients in the information exchange process? In this chapter we use the circuit of culture framework (du Gay et al., 1997) to investigate health info(r)mediation in six professions. Our analysis focuses primarily on how these professions represent the identities of practitioners and clients as health information is exchanged with or delivered to them.

Identifying, providing and/or discussing health information with patients or clients features prominently in the practice of nurses, general medical practitioners, social workers working in health settings, dieticians, pharmacists and librarians. This role, although variously expressed and described, is evident in the scope of practice statements of each profession. Such statements may be very broad, serving to extend an occupation's range of control in relation to other occupations (Winter, 1988). For example, the Canadian Medical Association (2000) claims a scope of practice that includes anything done under the supervision of a physician, while the American Nurses Association (2001) claims that nursing is whatever a nurse does. Within these two professions, info(r)mediary work is described as 'patient education'. In the scope of practice statements for social work, dietetics and pharmacy, health info(r)mediation activity is inferred, but the nature or extent of the professions' responsibility is not explicit. Only librarians represent info(r)mediary work as the primary focus of their professional practice.

To explore how info(r)mediation is understood in these professions, we examined the content of websites produced by Canadian, UK and US organizations that represent each group. In addition, we reviewed examples of professional curricula,[2] including course outlines, readings and texts that are concerned with practices relating to health information exchange. We also searched for references to info(r)mediary work in recent issues of English-language journals directed to practitioners. Finally, we looked to data gathered from research undertaken as part of the Action for Health project (see Acknowledgements) to describe the experiences of patients and clients who have participated in health information exchanges with members of these professional groups.

Health info(r)mediary work in the professions

General practice medicine

> The doctor we have now, we really don't agree with on much. I trust that he's very well educated and he knows his stuff, but he's not a good people person and he doesn't trust that we know what's good for us. He really, he is 'I am the doctor. I know', which just annoys me.
> (person living with HIV/AIDS [PHA])[3]

This patient has a poor opinion of his physician's ability to communicate information and is justified in expecting more. According to the Canadian Medical Association (2000: 3), a competent physician is expected to be a 'medical expert, communicator, scholar, collaborator, manager, health advocate and professional'. The role of 'communicator' positions physicians' info(r)mediary work in the context of a 'therapeutic relationship'. Competence in this role includes the ability to 'obtain and synthesize relevant history from patients, families and communities, to listen effectively, and to discuss appropriate information with patients, families and health care team members' (Canadian Medical Association, 2000: 10).

Medical educators in the UK and Canada recognize the need to improve physicians' ability to communicate. Their curricular materials for those entering the profession emphasize the importance of the patient interview as a means to build a relationship with a patient and to enhance the doctor's understanding of the patient's point of view, rather than simply as an information-gathering process driven by the physician

(Lussier and Richards, 2004; Silverman et al., 2005). Physician education materials stress that information-giving can contribute to positive health outcomes and is highly related to patient satisfaction, but explain that while most patients prefer more information and wish to be involved in shared decision making, some do not. They also recommend a variety of techniques to be used by physicians as they interact with patients and their families. The PHA quoted above might well have had a more positive view of his treatment and of his relationship with his doctor if the physician had used the techniques recommended in the contemporary medical curriculum.

Although most patients would probably be delighted to have access to physicians who use the practices recommended by Silverman et al., in health systems where physicians are paid by the procedure (as is the case in much of Canada and the United States), time limitations restrict their use. Indeed, although for most people physicians are still the most trusted source of health information (see Harris et al., 2006), patients repeatedly complain that physicians are rushed. For example, Wathen and Harris (2007) report that rural women who were interviewed about how they locate health information frequently commented on the limited time doctors spend with patients. According to one woman, 'Doctors are so overworked they don't have time to have friendly discussion with people.' Another said:

> [D]octors don't have a lot of time so you have to be very prepared. You have to go in with your questions and know exactly what information you're looking for. It's almost like you need to know the answers before you ask the questions. I find a lot of doctors tend to talk at you instead of with you.
>
> (Wathen and Harris, 2007)

In their professional literature, physicians' competence as 'communicators' is twinned with their expertise as 'scholars', with both practice competencies expected to contribute to their effectiveness in patient education (i.e. in their info(r)mediary work). For instance, the scholar physician is expected to 'develop, implement and monitor a personal continuing education strategy, to appraise critically sources of medical information, to facilitate learning of patients, house staff, students and other health professionals, and to contribute to development of new knowledge' (Canadian Medical Association, 2000: 10). In their roles as scholars, educators and communicators, physicians clearly represent themselves as health information experts *vis-à-vis* their patients (and other health care providers). While many patients are content to accept their physicians' expertise and leave it up to them to make medical decisions (see Henwood et al., 2003), some want a more active role in their own treatment or to talk with their physician about information they locate from other sources. Physicians may object to such input into the information exchange process, preferring a top-down model of info(r)mediation, the very approach that elicits complaints like that of the PHA cited above, or by a rural resident who observed that 'the "doctor is God" attitude is very unhelpful' (Harris et al., 2006).

The physician's role as information 'expert' is being embedded in the emerging practice of 'information therapy', in which physicians are encouraged to 'prescribe' information to their patients. According to Kemper and Mettler (2002: vii, viii), 'information is medicine' that 'can be prescribed, just like a pill', a service which, they argue, should be covered by 'reimbursement formulas'. Kemper and Mettler claim that information prescriptions supported by automated 'push' systems, such as targeted email messages to patients, provide a means by which physicians and health management organizations (especially in the US) can be compensated for specific instances of what they describe as 'patient education'. These emerging practices will further exacerbate tensions between physicians and those patients who want to be 'talked with' rather than 'talked at'.

Although physicians are expected to be scholars and experts, they don't necessarily produce the information they provide to their patients. Rather, physicians 'consume' information, some of which is produced by drug manufacturers through advertising in professional journals, in print materials supplied directly to them or through online courses available as part of their required continuing medical education. In addition, physicians rely increasingly on the internet to locate medical information (Martin, 2003; Henderson, 2005). However, because many patients also have ready access to internet-based health information, there is growing concern among some physicians over what Ahmad et al. (2006: 9) describe as 'Internet-generated "reversed" information asymmetry'. Increasingly, physicians are expected to respond to the material patients introduce into the health information exchange, a process some regard as problematic in their relationship with patients. According to Ahmad et al., physicians see the information that patients retrieve from the internet as adding 'a new interpretive role to their clinical responsibilities' and, while most feel 'obliged to carry out this new responsibility, the additional role was often unwelcome' (2006: 8). At present, there are no clear practice guidelines as to how this role should be performed and many physicians do not have the skills to 'undertake the contextualization and interpretation of such information' (Ahmad et al., 2006: 9).

For general practice physicians, info(r)mediary work is not represented as the neutral provision of information to patients, but rather as part of a process described as 'patient education'. By educating their patients, physicians expect to achieve improved patient outcomes (including compliance with treatments prescribed by the physician) and (in some cases) patient satisfaction. While two-way information exchange and relationship-building are advocated in the practice literature, time constraints may preclude effective communication and reinforce a one-way, top-down approach to information exchange, leaving patients feeling unheard. It remains to be seen whether patients' capacity to locate and retrieve health information on their own, independently of their doctors, will destabilize physicians' identity as 'experts' and/or if practices such as online information 'prescribing' will further contribute to patient alienation.

Social work

A woman living in a rural area described a social worker as her best source of health information.

> [S]he can refer me, she has information, she's a good facilitator. You can ask her for just about anything and she can direct you. If she doesn't know she finds out and calls you later. She's very, very good and she gives you the feeling that she's got all the time in the world to spend with you and I know her caseload is big. She's really the best.
> (Harris and Wathen, 2007)

According to the Canadian Association of Social Workers (2006), social workers 'help people develop their skills and their ability to use their own resources and those of the community'. Although this statement does not make explicit reference to info(r)mediation, generalist social work is usually represented as consisting of eight distinct roles – counsellor, educator, broker, case manager, mobilizer, mediator, facilitator and advocate (Karst-Ashman and Hull, 2006). Of these, the role of 'educator' – one who 'gives information and teaches skills' (Karst-Ashman and Hull, 2006: 25) – best captures the social worker's info(r)mediary responsibilities.

Like physicians, social workers do their info(r)mediary work in the context of a relationship with a client (or patient). However, while a physician's info(r)mediary work is most likely to be with individual patients, generalist social workers also work with couples, families, groups and communities. A basic component of this work is the interview, which is an opportunity for two-way communication to establish a relationship, confirm a purpose, use listening skills, gather information and offer help, which can include 'clarification, confrontation, interpretation, and providing information, suggestions and advice' (Kadushin, 1995: 1532), all components of what we would call info(r)mediation. Information exchange can occur at all stages of work with a client. In an 'intake' interview, for example, the social worker clarifies his or her purpose or role (Shulman, 2000: 127) and may exchange information and facilitate appropriate referrals (Johnson et al., 2000: 111). Info(r)mediation can also be embedded in treatment plans implemented over a number of weeks or months. Info(r)mediary work, therefore, is clearly a basic component of generalist social work practice.

Info(r)mediation related to health issues is most common in medical social work, one of the first social work specializations to be articulated by the profession in the US in the 1930s. This specialty was originally intended to 'augment the physician's treatment of patients by studying, reporting, and alleviating to the extent possible the patients' social problems that interfered with the plan for medical care' (Ross, 1995: 1365). As child welfare and income security programmes developed, this support role became less significant. However, two more roles emerged for medical social workers: discharge planning and patient education. In the former, the social worker serves as a liaison between the physician and community resources, organizing services so that the patient can safely leave hospital. The latter involves considerable info(r)mediation and was initially focused on patient compliance and intended to 'enlist cooperation with the medical treatment plan through patient education' (Ross, 1995: 1365). This concern with 'compliance' is more muted in contemporary statements about medical social work. As Ross explains, modern medical social work is concerned with 'helping people facing illness, trauma-related crises, or disability to understand and manage the psychosocial impact on their lives and on significant relationships and to make decisions and plan for the future' (1995: 1369).

Whether in generalist social work or medical social work practice, the positioning of clients (or patients) *vis-à-vis* the social worker is more egalitarian than that existing between physicians and patients. Indeed, the profession's ethical code emphasizes client 'self-determination' as a primary focus (Canadian Association of Social Workers, 2005). The social worker supports clients, helping them consider and/or cope with information relevant to their circumstances. For instance, the info(r)mediary work of medical social workers in hospital settings or in organizations focused on specific illnesses (such as HIV/AIDS or breast cancer) is often represented as 'psychoeducation'. This term denotes social work interventions that combine providing information and offering support to deal with the psychological and social impact of that information. Psychoeducation is used with clients and family members, individually and in groups, to help people and their families cope with a range of acute and chronic illnesses and their psychosocial consequences. To do this work, social workers are often responsible for producing pamphlets, posters and websites (Bella et al., 2005) for their client populations. However, even though employers have identified advanced information search skills and use of electronic resources as needed on the job (Canadian Association of Social Workers, 2000), these skills do not feature in social work curricula.

Overall, info(r)mediation within social work is part of a broadly defined helping process in which the client is seen to be self-determining. Social workers claim less expert knowledge than their colleagues in the medical profession.[4] While medical social workers are skilled in the interpersonal processes of info(r)mediation and helping people to address the psychosocial consequences of illness, they may lack the technical skills needed to keep up with the medical information involved in their practice and to update the materials they are expected to produce. Nevertheless, done well, health info(r)mediation by social work practitioners can be a very powerful experience for clients.

Nursing

Nurses and nurse practitioners are often on the front line as info(r)mediary workers. In the following example, a nurse practitioner who provides support to patients coping with a positive diagnosis of HIV infection explains how her clients' readiness for information varies.

> It could be that, yeah, they're here for an hour and a half, but then they're back again tomorrow or the next day for another hour, you know, and they're sort of just building on ... they've gone home with some information now, and they're going to have questions in two days' time again or they want to ... come back in.[5]

Info(r)mediary work is clearly central to and explicit in this nurse's practice. In Wathen and Harris' (2007) study of rural women's health information-seeking practices, one woman remarked that nurses 'are not good at diagnosing or explaining but they are very caring and they usu-ally help to calm you down'. Another explained that nurses 'give a lot more information ... it seems to be hands on, sort of applied, as opposed to theoretical and I think they're quite effective'. Others said that nurses, friends or family members are among the first people they turn to when they need medical advice.

Nursing has a long history of involvement in education, including both info(r)mediary work with individuals (such as the support described above) and instruction in group settings. In fact, Florence Nightingale devoted 'a large portion of her career to educating physicians, health offi-cials, and nurses about the importance of proper conditions' for health (Bastable, 1997: 5). Although much nursing practice falls under the supervision and even direction of physicians, education has persisted as a significant domain for autonomous nursing practice. The nurse's contemporary scope of practice includes 'direct patient care provider, *educator*, administrator, research, policy developer or other' (American Nursing Association, 2001; emphasis added).

Education is a central role for nurses within contemporary community health care systems. Public health nurses promote health as they teach in schools and elsewhere about matters such as sexuality (Kennedy, 2005). In community care settings, nurses, like social workers, understand patient education to include 'supporting' patients and families with chronic health conditions by facilitating and leading support groups and by providing information (Lawton et al., 2005). For example, nurses who specialize in supporting people affected by multiple sclerosis (MS) will:

> empower those affected by MS by providing information, support and advice about the condition from the time of diagnosis and throughout the disease spectrum. The MS specialist nurse is pivotal in providing a greater understanding of the condition and, by adopting a holistic, collaborative and coordinated approach can help those individuals, where possible, reach their goals of self-management.
>
> (MacLean and Russell, 2005: 755)

In nursing, patient education involves a 'process of assisting the patient to gain knowledge, skills and a value or attitude related to a health problem or for health promotion' (Stedman, 2005: 1093). The intent of patient education is often to facilitate informed consent by patients by providing 'accurate, complete and understandable informa-tion in a manner that facilitates informed judgment' as well as 'support and advice from knowledgeable nurses' (American Nursing Association,

2001). Nurses also educate patients who are being discharged, teaching them and their families how to manage the illness at home. This role has become more significant as health care cutbacks and new technologies result in earlier discharge from hospital (Bastable, 1997).

Contemporary nursing curricula include both communication skills and preparation for the nurse's role as educator (Bastable, 1997; Arnold and Boggs, 2003). Bastable sets out three approaches for understanding patient 'motivation' and 'compliance'. In the 'compliance' model, the nurse educator holds expert power and the patient complies from a position of dependency. In the 'adherence' model, the patient has more power, but still 'conforms' to expert expectations. In the third (and supposedly ideal) 'therapeutic alliance' model, power is shared equally between the patient and the health care provider. Bastable describes the therapeutic alliance model as the 'self-care' pole of the power continuum. However, the continuum does not include a pole where the patient is seen as autonomous and self-determining. This is an interesting exclusion, given the nursing profession's commitment to informed consent.

We found the nursing literature to be pragmatic and largely uncritical in adopting new information technologies, with nurses 'embracing' the new technology and 'e-nursing' (e.g. Auffrey, 2005). In one such project, nurses received 'just-in-time emails' reminding them of evidence-based practice standards for post-cardiac care which, according to Pezzin et al. (2005), resulted in improved patient understanding, clinical outcomes and adherence. Nurses' roles as health info(r)mediators have also been incorporated (and circumscribed) within government-sponsored telephone nurse advisory services, such as the Nurseline in British Columbia, Canada (see Balka and Butt, this volume), which provides the public with 24-hour access to nurses who use scripts to respond to inquiries and to provide advice.[6]

Dieticians and nutritionists[7]

> A mother who feared she might lose custody of her eight-year-old son unless he lost weight was allowed to keep the boy after striking a deal yesterday with social workers to safeguard his welfare.
>
> (Norfolk, 2007: 11)

This news article from the UK questions whether the child's obesity is the result of genetics, junk food or bad parenting, and goes on to explain that nutritionists and social workers plan to solve the problem through a contract with the child's mother, in which she agreed to adhere to a prescribed diet for her son. The mother's compliance is central to her continued custody of her child. In our review of their practice literature, we found that compliance with food and eating regimes is central to the practice of dieticians and explicit in their info(r)mediary work.

The food and nutrition field in general, and the dietetics profession in particular, originated in the academic discipline of home economics, a sister discipline to agricultural science (Maclean, 1994). The gendered division between the study of food production and food consumption resulted in a sense of inferiority for those working in 'home economics', and a persistent search for credibility for the discipline and its scientific base (Maclean, 1994), In contemporary practice, dieticians manage institutional food services, promote public health and counsel those for whom nutrition is an element of recovery. In the UK the profession's scope of practice covers the use of the science of nutrition to 'devise eating plans for patients to treat medical conditions' and to promote health by facilitating 'a positive change in food choices amongst individuals, groups and communities'.[8] Info(r)mediation is central to dieticians' efforts to improve people's food choices.

In acute care and extended care settings, dieticians manage food services for 'captive patients' and work to persuade patients to comply with a prescribed healthy diet. Good nutrition, for example, is significant in managing many common chronic conditions such as diabetes and hypertension, and included in the long-term management of HIV (Fenton, 2004). Like nurses, dieticians prepare patients for discharge by educating them about nutrition at home. According to Howard et al., 'a fundamental aspect of dietetic practice is the singular ability of the dietician to translate complex clinical nutritional concepts into simple everyday language coupled with acceptable strategies for implementing nutritional change' (1999: 380). Ideally, such information and advice are to be embodied in a 'nutrition care plan' developed by an interdisciplinary team, including the physician and other health care personnel, using a 'family centered approach' (Wessel et al., 2005).

Most materials about the professional practice of dieticians focus on persuading people (whether patients or members of the general public) to change their dietary practices to conform to the recommendations of experts. As in the newspaper story cited above, compliance is the goal. But, as dieticians learn in practice, lay people can ignore, refuse or fail to follow their guidance – a problem they describe as a 'knowledge deficit' on the part of patients (Hansen et al., 2003). Dieticians learn about interpersonal skills in courses similar to those in nursing and social work, and are introduced to social work literature on 'motivational interviewing' (Wahab, 2005). The language of 'patient' or 'client' self-determination, evident in the literatures of social work and nursing (at least in the latter in relation to 'informed consent') seem absent from the practice discourse of dieticians and nutritionists. Several studies suggest that people who fail to comply to prescribed diets lacked a sense of control over their lives, and would be more compliant if they felt more empowered (Fenton, 2004; Koelen and Lindstrom, 2005). We find this use of 'empowerment' an odd construct in the context of compliance with dietetic prescriptions.

Some in the dietetics field do describe a less expert-driven model of practice. Anderson (1998), for example, discusses a 'client-centred' model of the dietician as 'partner' rather than 'expert'; and Buchanan acknowledges that people make their own choices and suggests that trying to control people's behaviour in relation to food presents both ethical and practical problems. He recommends a 'humanistic approach' that is more tolerant of 'uncertainty in trying to aid people to improve their own skills of practical autonomy' (2004: 52). Similarly, Hansen et al. suggest that people's food choices are 'complex, situationally sensitive expressions of their personal value system' (2004: 120) and calls for a more contextualized understanding of people's perceptions of risk related to food. Others outside the field suggest changing the environment rather than individual behaviour to address problematic food choices. For instance, the American Academy of Pediatrics recommended reducing juvenile diabetes by removing soft drink dispensers from schools (Committee on School Health, 2004).

Like nurses, dieticians are attracted to newer technologies. They develop materials embodying their expertise (Savage and Auld, 2006) and in the US can access web-based teaching materials related to national dietary guidelines (Kendall, 2006). Dieticians are also advised to use the web to develop tools to support clinical decision making and computer simulations for training (Winkler, 2005). The internet is regarded as a potentially powerful tool, both for disseminating information to the general public and for providing nutrition counselling to individuals (e.g. Verheijden et al., 2005; Fernandez-Celemin et al., 2006).

Dieticians, like nurses and physicians, represent their info(r)mediary work as 'patient education'; they position themselves as experts who rely on and convey information derived from a specialized, scientific knowledge base. Although their code of ethics requires dietetics practitioners to provide sufficient information for clients and others to make their own informed decisions (American Dietetic Association, 1999), the right to self-determination seems absent from the practice literature. Dieticians appear to share a belief, even a professional ideology, that if information drawn from their domain of expertise is presented in the context of scientific 'proof', their 'clients', whether individual patients or members of the public, will comply with prescribed diets and correct their 'bad' eating habits. The dietician appears to assume that 'talking at' patients from a position of scientific expertise is the basis of effective info(r)mediary work.

Pharmacy

Pharmacists' scope of practice combines up-to-date, technical knowledge with the ability to work with people and good communication skills. The profession's ethical code is explicit about pharmacists' responsibility for info(r)mediary work. They must 'provide their patients with information that is truthful, accurate and understandable so that the patients are able to make informed choices about their health care' (Nova Scotia College of Pharmacists, 2007). Patients are often confused by inconsistencies between what their doctors have to say about the benefits of certain drugs and how pharmacists describe the same medications and their potential side-effects (Semchuk, 2004). The approach taken by pharmacists is preferred by many of the patients or clients. Indeed, as the following comments suggest, Wathen and Harris (2007) found that that rural women who were interviewed about their health information seeking often praised their pharmacists:

I find the pharmacist very helpful. If I have a question about a condition or medicine, I find they are extremely helpful and they seem to almost be a substitute for the doctors because the doctors aren't available.

And,

Pharmacy guys are really good at explaining.

Like dieticians, pharmacists are familiar with non-compliant patients. For instance, only about half those with chronic conditions such as hypertension continue to take prescribed life-extending medications, a situation unimproved over 25 years (Semchuk, 2004). However, unlike the approach to clients that characterizes dietetic practice, the info(r)mediary work of pharmacists is directed to information accuracy and patient self-determination rather than compliance. What pharmacists call 'patient counselling' involves providing technical information about the name of a drug, the reasons for taking it, the time for taking it and its potential side-effects. Pharmacists' expertise has been recognized in a recent announcement by the government of Ontario of a new programme for citizens who are taking three or more medications for chronic conditions. The programme entitles these patients to 30 minutes a year to consult their pharmacist. According to the Ontario Minister of Health, 'we have a lot of brain power invested in pharmacists'.[9]

Despite the centrality of info(r)mediary work in pharmacy practice, communication skills are not consistently central to pharmacy education. For instance, while communications skills were part of a required first year course in one curriculum we reviewed, in another it was a fifth year elective. This contrasts with the emphasis in professional curricula in medicine, nursing, social work and nutrition where these skills are explicitly and consistently embedded. On the other hand, pharmacy curricula do emphasize technological issues, albeit largely uncritically. For instance, one introductory pharmacy practice text describes the extent to which pharmacists use new information technologies. Software facilitates and even automates the dispensing process, presumably thereby releasing more time for pharmacists to interact with patients. Technology permits more patient screening at the pharmacy, and the internet is represented as a tool that enables pharmacists to communicate with physicians and to locate more up-to-date information about the drugs they dispense (Bowman et al., 2000; West et al., 2000). Pharmacists' associations also enthuse about the emerging field of pharmacy health informatics and advocate adoption of new information technology such as 'e-prescribing' and the electronic health record (MacDonald et al., 2005; Canadian Pharmacists Association, 2006). Pharmacists have also been involved in the production of new technologies. For example, pilot projects have successfully networked pharmacists with physicians and patients (Chan et al., 2004), and a Canadian web portal gives primary care practitioners 'point-of-care access to current, evidence-based, Canadian drug and therapeutic information to support best practices' (Canadian Pharmacists Association, 2007: 1). An association website also provides patient-friendly leaflets and materials directed to children to teach lay people about prescription drugs, and pharmacists can serve the public by 'refuting misinformation or by reframing the information' found on the web (Ives et al., 2000: 53).

While the profession has welcomed these benefits of technology, the transnational nature of the internet has also been problematic. For example, some Canadian pharmacists use e-commerce to sell prescriptions to customers in other countries, particularly the US.

Increasingly, Canadian pharmacies are using the Internet to market their services for dispensing of prescription drugs for export to citizens of the United States and other countries. Some others use a "store front" intermediary or other means to market their services. This trade is now estimated at over $1 billion annually. Much of this growth is driven by the difference in the price of pharmaceuticals between Canada and the US, coupled with the fact that many American seniors do not have a comprehensive drug benefits plan.

(Canadian Pharmacists Association, 2004: 1)

The Canadian Pharmacists Association argues that cross-border prescription drug sales endanger patients and emphasize the significance of their own info(r)mediary role. 'Face-to-face communication between patients and pharmacists builds a relationship ... [that is] essential for medication management and to ensure that patients understand how to use their drugs safely and effectively' (Canadian Pharmacists Association, 2004: 2). In cross-border prescription sales, the pharmacist has no relationship with the patient and care may be compromised. They also cite the Canadian Medical Association's reminder that no doctor should sign a prescription without personally assessing the patient and call for the government to ban the exporting of drugs from Canadian pharmacies. In contrast, the code of ethics for pharmacists in the UK requires only that 'on-line' pharmaceutical care be of the same high quality as face-to-face service on pharmacy premises and suggests that on-line care may be in the interest of the patient (Royal Pharmaceutical Society of Great Britain, 2004: 3).

Of all the health professions discussed, pharmacy is most concerned with the accuracy of information. Like physicians, pharmacists claim independent expertise, and keep that expertise up to date through use of newer information technologies. Although they may use the term 'counselling' to describe info(r)mediary work with customers, descriptions of such counselling suggest it is comparatively neutral information exchange outside the context of a therapeutic relationship. Also, with an explicit responsibility to address side-effects, pharmacists appear to be less wholehearted about compliance than other health professions and more firmly committed to embedding their practice in emerging technologies.

Librarianship

Of all the professions we consider in this chapter, only librarianship makes info(r)mediation (usually described as 'reference' work) central to its practice. As the following description shows, this profession is being transformed by technology.

> The traditional concept of a library is being redefined from a place to access paper records or books to one that also houses the most advanced media, including CD-ROM, the Internet, virtual libraries, and remote access to a wide range of resources. Consequently, librarians, or information professionals, increasingly are combining traditional duties with tasks involving quickly changing technology. Librarians assist people in finding information and using it effectively for personal and professional purposes. Librarians must have knowledge of a wide variety of scholarly and public information sources and must follow trends related to publishing, computers, and the media in order to oversee the selection and organization of library materials. Librarians manage staff and develop and direct information programs and systems for the public, to ensure that information is organized in a manner that meets users' needs.
>
> (Bureau of Labor Statistics, 2006–7)

In this context, librarians provide user services, technical services and administrative services. Within user services, providing reference service (or helping patrons find the information they need), is a core professional role which involves

> analyzing users' needs to determine what information is appropriate, as well as searching for, acquiring, and providing the information. The job also includes an instructional role, such as showing users how to access information. For example, librarians commonly help users navigate the Internet in search of relevant information.
>
> (Bureau of Labor Statistics, 2006–7)

Within the more specialized field of medical/health librarianship, info(r)mediation includes a major role in producing and organizing health information in print collections and electronic form, and helping people access these resources. Librarians also produce 'finding aids' and have worked to produce consumer health portals, such as the UK's online consumer health information service, NHS Direct,[10] and Canada's health information portal, the Canadian Health Network.[11] Librarians also manage the United States National Library of Medicine, the world's largest medical library that produces, among other things, the well-known online databases Medline (for scientists and physicians) and Medline Plus (for lay people).[12]

Librarians are expected to play an educating or 'instructional' role in their work with clients (who are usually described as 'users' or 'patrons'). However, while librarians help people find information, unlike the health care professionals described above, they do not have a therapeutic context for their work. The librarian's expertise is in the organization and retrieval of information, an expertise which includes familiarity with new and emerging information technologies and a leadership role in designing information systems in which these technologies are used. While 'interpretation' is a responsibility that is expected of other professional health info(r)mediaries, such as medical social workers who provide psychoeducation, when librarians facilitate access to information, the interpretation of information is explicitly precluded from their role, particularly when it comes to legal and health information, although as we see in the next chapter, in practice, avoiding 'interpretation' can be a challenge for library staff. As a result, the idea of 'compliance' is absent from librarianship's discourse, except where library users are encouraged to use librarian-developed tools or finding aids, such as catalogues or classification systems, to locate materials on their own.

Representing info(r)mediary work in the professions

We began this chapter by quoting Nettleton and Burrows (2003), who suggest that the widespread availability of health information via the internet is changing the nature of the health information exchange. They point out that medical knowledge is now accessible to lay people and is no longer produced and regulated solely by experts. The info(r)mediary practices of all the professions we have discussed in this chapter have been affected by the emergence of internet-based health information. The librarian, for example, plays a central role in the actual production and management of health information systems. Librarians build the collections, write the finding aids and help the people who visit or phone the reference desk. Health librarians also construct systems used by members of the health professions to access current information about illness and treatment. To a large degree, the future effectiveness of the info(r)mediary work of the five health professions outlined here (medicine, nursing, social work, pharmacy and dietetics) will ultimately depend on foundations built by the librarians and information technology specialists who produce and manage health information systems and help others to use them.

Each of the six professions we have described in this chapter engage in health info(r)mediary work. However, as we have shown, within

Providing Information ::	Librarian; Pharmacist
Patient Education ::	Dietician; Nurse; Physician
Psychoeducation ::	Social Worker

Figure 2.1   Contrasting representations of professional info(r)mediary work

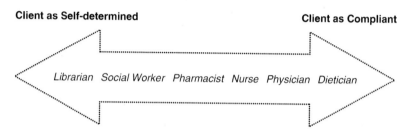

Figure 2.2   Representations of the recipients of info(r)mediary work

the professions there are different understandings of that work. At one pole, some professions position their info(r)mediary responsibilities as the neutral provision of information, with concern for accuracy (in the case of pharmacists), and without judgement or interpretation of the information (in the case of librarians) (see Figure 2.1).

In their practice, of the six professions, librarians most closely operate as what Latour (2005) describes as 'intermediaries', as they 'transport meaning' without 'transformation'. On the other hand, dieticians, nurses and physicians use the term 'patient education' to describe their info(r)mediary work and position it in the context of a therapeutic relationship through which they impart information as 'experts', that is, in Latour's terms, they actively 'mediate', often 'transforming' the information they pass on to others. For social workers, info(r)mediary work is threaded throughout encounters with those they help, and in the context of medical social work encompasses psychoeducation to help people both understand information about their condition and deal with its psychic and social consequences.

The six professions also have contrasting representations of the person who receives the information (Figure 2.2). The librarian has a 'patron' and the retail pharmacist has a 'customer'. The social worker works with a 'client' and the nurse, physician and dietician all work with a 'patient'. Embedded in these contrasting terms are the professions' differing positions related to compliance and self-determination. This concern ranges

Knowledge Broker   **Independent Expert**

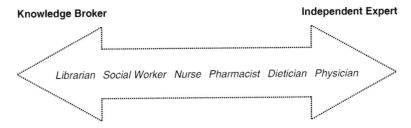

Figure 2.3 Representation of professions' expert knowledge

from preoccupation with compliance (for the dieticians) to its irrelevance (for the librarian). The concern with compliance also persists for medicine and nursing, often accompanied by the assumption that information is all that will be required for a patient to conform to a diet or exercise plan or to take medication as prescribed. Although the naivety of this assumption is noted in both the pharmacy and dietetics literatures, the pursuit of compliance persists.

Thirdly, the six professions differ in the extent to which they represent themselves as having independent expertise, in contrast to those professions who represent themselves as knowledge brokers (Figure 2.3). We found dieticians to be most emphatic about their independent scientific expertise. Pharmacists and physicians, too, present themselves as experts, but rely extensively on sources of information prepared and organized for them by others. Nurses, and to a lesser extent social workers, gather information from others and are responsible for its presentation so that it can be understood by patients and clients. They produce information materials, but usually with derived information. Finally, the librarian is the knowledge broker in purest form, responsible for organizing and retrieving information and for helping others to find the information they need and want.

In terms of emerging information technologies, practitioners in all the health professions consume internet-based health information, although to varying extents. However, they have done much less to respond to the public's growing access to internet-based health information. Physicians rely on internet-based technologies to update their own expert knowledge, but may be impatient with patients who bring this information to the doctor–patient interview. As a result, tensions grow between physician and patient. Pharmacists are energetic users and promoters of internet-based health information and pride themselves in providing accurate and unbiased information to patients. Patients seem to value their pharmacist's advice, but in most systems patient counselling is not yet a chargeable service (the new initiative in Ontario being an exception). Nursing has accepted the opportunities provided by new information technologies to extend the reach of patient education, but their face-to-face practice is not generally framed in terms of interpreting information that patients may gain from the internet. Social workers engage in health info(r)mediation, particularly in health settings, and through psychoeducation may help people cope with the implications of health information about an illness. However, professional education and continuing education have done little to help social workers to use and interpret (and to help others interpret) internet-based health information. Of all the professions discussed here, dieticians are the ones most convinced of the value of their own expertise, believing that their information is a powerful tool in changing unhealthy eating behaviours. However, professions that rely heavily on the 'expert' role in health info(r)mediation, such as dietetics, and who persist in 'talking at' their patients, may be the most vulnerable to the changes wrought by the democratizing effects of the internet.

Health info(r)mediary work pervades the practice of the six professions described in this chapter. However, as we have shown, these professions vary in their representation of that work and in their representation of the person who is its focus. The nature of this health info(r)mediation is changing as each profession responds, and responds differently, to the opportunities provided by new information technologies. The demands of this work are also changing as lay persons learn to locate, retrieve, exchange and even produce their own health information (or opinions). More and more, clients and patients will expect health professionals to help them to retrieve, understand and interpret internet-based health information. They want professionals to talk 'with' them rather than 'at' them, to discuss and help them interpret and evaluate information from various sources. Many will want help to make their own decisions about health issues, rather than being on the receiving end of a top-down exchange intended to secure compliance. As the internet democratizes access to health care information, more egalitarian info(r)mediary practices will be expected of practitioners in the health professions.

Notes

1. The title of a song by Harry Nilsson.
2. We thank the following: Jonathan Silverman, Associate Clinical Dean, Clinical Skills Unit, School of Clinical Medicine, Addenbrooke's Hospital,

Cambridge; Jacqui Gingras, Assistant Professor, School of Nutrition, Ryerson University, Toronto, Ontario; Lynda Bentley Poole, Chair, BScN programme, McMaster University, Hamilton, Ontario.

3. This quote is drawn interviews with people living with HIV/AIDS (PHAs), their family members, friends and health care providers as part of the 'Rural HIV/AIDS Information Networks Project' funded by the Canadian Institutes of Health Research.

4. While health issues may be addressed in undergraduate elective courses in the social work curriculum, preparation for medical social work is usually through specialized graduate work.

5. This quote is drawn from one of the interviews in the 'Rural HIV/AIDS Information Networks Project'.

6. http://www.bchealthguide.org/nurseline.stm.

7. Dietician is the title for a registered professional. A dietician will be a nutritionist, but a nutritionist will not necessarily be a dietician.

8. http://www.hpc-uk.org/aboutregistration/professions/dieticians/index/asp

9. http://ca.news.yahoo.com/s/capress/070717/health/health_pharmacists_drug_consultations.

10. http://www.nhsdirect.nhs.uk/.

11. http://www.canadian-health-network.ca/.

12. http://www.nlm.nih.gov/medlineplus/.

3

Health Intermediaries? Positioning the Public Library in e-Health Discourse

Flis Henwood, Roma Harris, Samantha Burdett and Audrey Marshall

Much existing policy and literature on public libraries and health information seeking is framed, implicitly at least, within 'e-health' discourse, which understands health information as empowering and the internet as a tool for accessing that information. In this discourse, public libraries are understood as key intermediaries of health information, offering both specialist services in information retrieval and free access to the internet for consumer-citizens who are active and responsible information seekers. Through an exploration of the practices involved in supporting health information-seeking practices in the public library context,[1] this chapter analyses how understanding e-health discourse can help us make sense of the specific sociotechnical configuration set up in the public library to support these practices. The analysis draws on the circuit of culture model (du Gay et al., 1997) to explore and understand how the public library is represented in e-health discourse; what identities or 'subject positions' are produced for both library staff and users within this discourse and the relationship between production and consumption activities, what we might think of as the mediating processes involved in e-health practices in the public library.

Our approach to studying representation here is a constructivist one, which draws on the discursive approach associated with Foucault's concept of discourse, which involves both language/talk and practice. As Hall argues, for Foucault discourse is:

> a group of statements which provide a language for talking about – a way of representing the knowledge about – a particular topic at a particular historical moment...Discourse is about the production of knowledge through language. But...since all social practices entail

meaning, and meanings shape and influence what we do – our conduct – all practices have a discursive element.

(Hall, 1992: 291, cited in Hall, 1997: 44)

Foucault is not arguing that things have no real, material existence in the world, but that nothing has any meaning outside discourse (Foucault, 1972). Thus, the 'public library' can be understood as having no fixed meaning; rather, its meaning is given in discourse and there may well be contested meanings in circulation. In this chapter we argue that, in e-health discourse, the public library has come to represent universal access to information and, through this, the empowerment of user-citizens. What the public library and the internet 'mean' can be understood through the discourse of e-health and we can begin to tease out these meanings through both the statements made about them and the practices associated with them – what we think of as the wider sociotechnical configurations of e-health found in the public library.

Another important idea of Foucault's relevant to our use of discourse is his understanding of the relationship between knowledge and power. Power is understood not as top-down and repressive but as circulating, deployed and organized through a net-like organization (Foucault, 1980: 98). Knowledge is inextricably linked to relations of power because it is always applied to the regulation of social conduct or practice. In modern societies, power operates not through coercion and direct control, but through the creation of 'expert knowledges' which serve to channel or constrain thinking and action (Peterson and Lupton, 1996: xii). Insofar as public libraries are engaged in the mediation of such knowledge, how should their intermediary role be understood?

Linked to this understanding of power is Foucault's 'regimes of truth' idea. A 'regime of truth' is not the same as something being true, but can be understood as the practices that follow from a particular understanding of the world. Thus, even though it may not be 'true' that e-health interventions in the public library empower individuals, if everyone believes it to be so and specific sociotechnical configurations are implemented in support of that truth/knowledge, this becomes a 'regime of truth' and has real consequences for both staff and users in the public library context. It is these beliefs and their consequences that we explore below.

The circuit of culture approach also suggests that we need to examine the social identities associated with particular cultural forms and practices. Again adopting a Foucauldian approach, we understand identity in the context of discourse. For Foucault, the 'subject' is not pre-existing, but is 'produced in discourse' in two main ways. First, the discourse produces subjects, namely figures who personify the particular forms of knowledge which the discourse produces such as 'informed patients' or 'informed consumers'; second, the discourse produces 'subject positions' from which its knowledge and meaning make most sense (Hall, 1997). The analysis below examines the subject positions taken up by both staff and users of the public library in the context of their engagement in e-health practices.

Finally, the circuit of culture approach also suggests that we need to examine the production and consumption activities associated with cultural forms and practices. Questions we explore in this context include: How does the internet in particular figure in the production and consumption of health information in the public library? How do both staff and users interact with the internet to find health information? What do such sociotechnical practices mean for how the process of health info(r)mediation is understood in a public library context?

A Foucauldian approach is taken by Hand (2005), who explores perceptions of internet access in UK public libraries in the context of debates about self-education and empowerment. Hand highlights emerging conjunctions and disjunctions between government policy; library–institutional discourses, interests and strategies; and the everyday practices of citizens in the context of such access. Hand argues that whereas government policy discourse positions internet access in public libraries as supporting e-democracy and active citizenship, public library discourse positions the internet as an information retrieval tool, and users position it largely as a communication medium. Hand's analysis is useful in that in reminds us that:

> the internet is not a unitary technology that can simply be 'inserted' in intermediary sites ... What the internet is, how people 'come to it', and what its 'effect' will be depend on its ongoing cultural relocation, as different configurations of material and immaterial elements are combined to accomplish specific operations.
>
> (Hand, 2005: 385)

In this chapter, we draw on Foucault's notion of discourse and his understandings of knowledge/power to reflect on the sociotechnical configurations which constuite e-health in a public library context. Our argument is that the particular social, cultural and organizational practices we observed can be understood as part of e-health discourse, which promotes the idea of the informed health care consumer, who, sometimes with the help of library staff, accesses and uses health information to empower him- or herself. However, while key actors (managers, staff and users) do at times embody these understandings, in their statements and their practices there is also some very clear resistance to this dominant discourse which, if explored and exploited, could result in the emergence of a more progressive model for library service development, one that can support the emergence of more active, critical and engaged citizen-users rather than neoliberal consumer-users.

e-Health discourse and the public library

e-Health discourse, when applied in the context of public or consumer health information, can be understood as combining elements of two other dominant discourses of the late modern period: 'the new public health' (Peterson and Lupton, 1996) and 'e-society'.[2] In the developing critique of consumerism in 'Western' health care systems, several commentators have charted the shift from 'welfarist' to 'neoliberal' politics in health care that both characterized the last two decades of the twentieth century and set a new paradigm for health service delivery and organization for the twenty-first century. It is claimed that this shift is characterized by a changing conception of the self, from 'patient' to 'client' or 'consumer', a shift from passive to active subject or citizen. This new, active consumer of health care shows a capacity for independent decision-making, and a readiness to put information to use (Brock, 1995: 158–9; cited in Henderson and Peterson, 2002: 2).

Peterson and Lupton argue that the 'new public health' (NPH) is essentially a modernist project and, in the public health field, experts assist in the process of 'self-governance' through the advice they offer and through promoting institutions that facilitate 'healthy' choices (1996: xiii), an idea that, as discussed in the previous chapter, has apparently been embraced with enthusiasm by dieticians. Peterson and Lupton point out that epidemiological knowledge in particular has been applied to pursue the objectives of the NPH. Epidemiological knowledge plays a key role in the construction of 'truth' about disease, risk factors and categories of 'at risk' subjects (1996: xiii) and has remained dominant in NPH discourse even though its 'facts' are frequently disputed, by experts and non-experts alike.

Another key aspect of the NPH is the way in which there appears to be a 'duties' discourse alongside the 'rights' discourse. Baudrillard (1998) argues that consumption has become institutionalized not as a right or pleasure, but as a 'duty' of the modern citizen, and that consumption becomes a basis for a sense of self and identity. This idea is manifested in the NPH discourse and to some extent in health more generally, where we can find elements of compulsion surrounding the exercise of choice where, as Henderson and Petersen argue, '[t]he "good consumer" of health care is compelled to make choices, to exhibit appropriate "information seeking" behaviour, and to behave in certain prescribed ways (consulting "relevant" expertise, taking the "right" medicine, engaging in personal risk management, and so on)' (2002: 3).

There are clear parallels between the NPH and e-society discourse. In e-society discourse, there is a set of neoliberal assumptions about the progressive nature of new technologies and the way in which they can support greater freedoms and choices among individuals and communities. Flowing from these assumptions is a focus on the digital divide and an associated set of 'rights' to access to information and communication technologies (ICTs). Furthermore, there is also a powerful 'duties discourse', a set of 'imperatives' to take up the opportunities provided by the new technologies. To be a 'good' citizen in the e-society, one must be an e-citizen. In this scenario, non-users become a problem waiting to be fixed and the possibility of voluntary non-use is barely entertained (for exceptions, see Wyatt et al., 2002; Selwyn, 2003). Similarly, we see a focus on making the technologies accessible and usable rather than useful, despite the fact that the latter is likely to be a more significant predictor of acceptability (Davis et al., 1989).

Finally, with respect to learning, e-society discourse promotes the development of skills and competences, with training in ICTs being the framework for learning. In contrast, a more constructivist perspective would emphasize learning about ICTs and the development of a critical e-literacy. Although the more common term 'e-literacy' appears to go further than the previously popular term 'IT literacy', emphasizing the need to learn not just the technology but the kinds of e-services now available to those with access to ICTs (e-government services as well as banking, shopping, health, and so on), it still appears to be a market-driven model (Cushman and Klecun, 2005). A more critical e-literacy would go much further and include the ability to question, analyse and evaluate both technologies and the information and communication flows and content that different technologies enable. This idea is closer to some notions of advanced media literacy (Livingstone, 2003; OFCOM, 2005). The analysis in this chapter raises questions about the kinds of information and IT or e-literacy being promoted in the context of e-health practices in the public library context.

If e-health discourse can be understood as combining elements of the new public health and e-society discourses, how are public libraries positioned in relation to these discourses? In the health area, government policy in the UK (and elsewhere) is increasingly promoting the notion of informed choice and greater patient and public involvement in health care decision-making (Department of Health, 2001, 2004b). New approaches to the management of chronic diseases include the development of self-care strategies that involve individuals taking on greater responsibilities for themselves, their families and their communities (Department of Health, 2004c, 2005). Universal access to quality health information and ICTs is seen as a resource that is crucial to the success of this new approach to health service delivery. In this context, information provider services, such as public libraries, are understood as important intermediaries linking information resources with the health information needs of individuals and local communities. The Department of Health paper *Better Information, Better Choices, Better Health*, in discussing how to improve access to health information in the local community, suggests that local health care organizations 'may wish to consider how to reach the public in everyday non-NHS environments, for example, in supermarkets, pharmacies, schools *and libraries*' (2004a; emphasis added).

Public libraries are also positioned as key change agents within e-society discourse which links internet access to notions of digital citizenship, without the mechanism by which the two are linked ever being fully spelt out. Indeed, the UK's People's Network initiative, launched in 2000, which set out to connect all public libraries to the internet and provide ICT skills development among library staff, claimed staff would be able to play a central role in supporting 'digital citizenship' among their users. £120 million was spent providing broadband access to the internet in over 4,000 public libraries and training approximately 40,000 library staff so that they could deliver a range of ICT services expected of a modern library. By 2003, 10 per cent of all internet users accessed the internet from a public library, compared with just 3 per cent in 2001 (Sommerland et al., 2004). But how far is digital citizenship advanced by the provision of internet access in public spaces such as libraries? Apart from the internet terminals themselves, what needs to be in place before this can happen? In this chapter, we explore this question through a focus on health information and e-health resources. Our key question becomes: What sociotechnical configurations can best support the development of an active, engaged and critical healthy citizen as opposed to a more passive and dutiful informed health care consumer?

The literature of Library Studies (or Library Science) has begun to address such issues, if not always explicitly. There is only a very small body of research that explicitly examines the experiences of library staff supporting health information seekers, but what does exist suggests a debate has started about their role in this regard. Borman and McKenzie (2005), for example, have documented library staff's accounts of the reference transaction with respect to health enquiries and found that staff described this work in terms of 'barriers' and 'counter-strategies', suggesting that there are areas of conflict to be resolved in this encounter. Similarly, Kouame et al. (2005) suggest that perceptions of library staff and users regarding the role libraries should play in supporting health information enquiries can differ and that there is a need for better understanding and clarity on both sides. A key question here concerns the boundaries of librarians' knowledge and expertise in supporting health information enquiries. Library staff will have expertise in information retrieval and increasingly in internet use, but they may not have the specialist knowledge to support library users in relation to specific health enquiries.

A study by Dewdney et al. (1991) described the kinds of problems librarians encounter in the process of answering both legal and health enquiries. They suggested some ways in which public librarians might become more effective in their role as 'distributors of consumer information' in the context of the growth of consumer movements and the challenge to the traditionally powerful professions of law and medicine. This point links the library-based studies to the wider debate about the alleged shifts in power and responsibility that are said to characterize contemporary health care practice. How should and can public libraries support the shift towards the more 'informed patient' (Henwood et al., 2003; Kivits, 2004) or 'reflexive health care consumer' (Hardey, 2004; Nettleton et al., 2004)? One area of concern covered in the literature is the extent to which librarians can and should engage in evaluations or critical appraisal of health information found on behalf of users. Some commentators (Crespo, 2004; Kovacs, 2004) have promoted the idea of evaluation as a key component of library service support for health information seeking, but Allcock (2000) and later Kenyon and Casini (2002) have drawn attention to the liability and ethical issues raised when public librarians direct library users towards health information resources. The study on which the following analysis draws investigated the expectations and experiences of library staff and users in relation to such evaluation and appraisal work and our analysis will explore how libraries are positioned to support the growth of consumer movements and the so-called 'challenge' to traditional forms of authority, such as medicine.

Sociotechnical configurations of e-health in the public library

The city centre library in which the study took place opened in spring 2005, just a year before our research began. Several structural and organizational changes were implemented by the library service when the library opened. First, the library adopted an explicitly 'self-service' approach to service delivery, with self-service issue, renewal and return of books. Second, there would no longer be a separate reference section; instead, the reference collection was integrated into the main collection. Although there was still an enquiry desk, it covered all enquiries, was located on the first floor (and was not clearly signposted either on the ground floor or the first floor) and was always very busy. There were two staff on the enquiry desk at any one time (a professional librarian and a library assistant) and each had access to the library catalogues and the internet. Enquiry desk staff did not carry out what might be understood as a traditional 'reference interview', in health or other areas, as time spent with each user was limited to 10 minutes (with all other enquiries being categorized as 'research' and charged for or referred to another suitable information provider, as appropriate). The library's IT centre was located in a separate room and most terminals had to be booked. (A few were available on a first-come, first-served basis, but time on these was limited to 15 minutes.) There were a few internet terminals located in the main library area, but these were also time-limited. Technical assistance in operating the equipment was available, but no specific help in information searching was available to those choosing to use the internet.

One of the managers of the service linked this self-service organization explicitly to notions of choice and empowerment:

> We are trying to empower the users (or whatever the phrase is) to give people choices of what they want to do. So if they don't want to talk to a member of staff then they can come in and they can return their books, issue their books, collect their reservations on a PC without necessarily having to queue up.
>
> (Manager 2)

He went on to explain what happens if a user does approach the enquiry desk:

> There isn't much time for enquiry desk staff to do more research-intensive questions. I think we would normally say a maximum of

10 minutes for enquiry and if they can deal with them in less time then so much the better ... At the enquiry desk we might provide sort of short answers to questions, but then we would normally channel people to the resources that they can find out themselves.

(Manager 2)

For the most part, users seem to have embraced the library's self-service/self-help model. One user commented, 'If you had a problem you should try and sort it out yourself before you go and start asking for help from other people' (User 10). However, some library users' responses suggest that their adoption of the self-service model may have more to do with necessity than preference. The time issue and not being sure about what they could expect from staff were both mentioned in this regard: 'I'm always in a rush so if there's a queue I won't ... I'll just get stressed trying to find it on my own. ... but if there's someone free I will ask' (User 6).

Staff also appeared to be concerned about the shift to a self-service model of delivery and its impact on both their work and the experience of users. As can be seen from the quotation below, information technology and the internet are understood as part and parcel of the self-service delivery model:

I personally think they've thrown the baby out with the bathwater ... they've actually forgotten what libraries are about ... I mean with people in it, physical human beings who as well as helping people with IT technology, who actually know what they're talking about can give that sort of advice across a whole range of subjects ... there's no need for us, IT services replaced it all.

(Staff Member 1)

In reflecting on how users engaged with the public library in the context of health information seeking, staff drew on e-health discourse to position users as good, informed patients or consumers:

I think people's attitude to health has changed in that they feel more in control, more aware that they are responsible, hopefully more aware that they are responsible both for their mental and physical health, all these programmes on TV for instance, all these magazine articles, you know, if you smoke and drink and eat rubbish foods then they're going to suffer ... So, it's up to you to do something about it. You can't just go to your doctor and say 'cure me', that's ridiculous. Well, I suppose there are still some people who [*laugh*] work on that basis, but hopefully our role would be to give people information, whichever way was suitable for their needs at the time and encourage them to, you know, look at their lifestyle.

(Staff Member 12)

Also consistent with e-health discourse, staff positioned themselves first and foremost as mediators in the sense of go-betweens, linking users who have information needs with appropriate information sources: '[our role] is to find the answer ... to match the information they require or the help they require or the health information or website address, whatever, just to answer somebody's inquiry to whatever level, whatever depth needed' (Staff Member 2). This depiction of the librarian's intermediary role is consistent with the positioning of the profession on the 'know-ledge broker' end of the continuum of expertise described by Bella et al. (this volume). However, the actual performance of this role often proves to be difficult, especially in health enquiries, where the linked needs for expressing care and giving time operated as constraints on this simple go-between role:

There is something emotional about somebody coming in and because it is personal to them. A lot of the time to be able to find the right information they do need to give you a bit of information [about] what is going on and you tend to find about the operation that they had, and headaches they have been getting, or the fact that they have just been diagnosed with cancer. It makes it more personal. You have to give that little bit more, do you not, on the enquiry desk.

(Staff Member 15)

While some users, at some points, also positioned themselves in line with this thinking, it is clear that they seek real interaction, not just a simple connection to resources:

I suppose I'm sort of a bit of a child, I expect them to find the answers if I ask them something. ... I left there really thinking ... 'It's not something that affects her directly, she doesn't really care.' I think she gave me about 8 minutes of her time.

(User 5)

What's more important is that you feel that they're genuinely helping you, rather than pointing over their shoulder toward a particular aisle.

> It's all to do with that moment with interaction, which is what gives you your final opinion on the librarians.
>
> (User 14)

Thus both staff and users express, and at the same time resist, the notion of the self-serving library user supported by staff who merely connect people who have 'information needs' with reliable and relevant resources. Health enquiries, perhaps because they are so often concerned with personal and intimate issues, seem to require a more engaged and caring approach, a model of interaction that might not be best supported by a self-help model of service delivery.

These kinds of relational issues are, we might argue, exacerbated by the presence of the internet in the health enquiry. Our survey of library users showed that while many are internet users and do use it to seek health information, not all are convinced of its reliability or usefulness. Similar to what has been reported elsewhere (e.g. Harris and Wathen, 2007), some of the library users find the information available via the internet overwhelming or frightening, do not trust the information they find and/or prefer to receive important information about their health from another person or from what they regard as more authoritative sources, such as books:

> I hate the internet. ... I can never find anything I want ... it's not like a book where you can just look down in the index, find the section you want, flip to it; you have to go through every damn thing first to find the one that you want ... Books you can keep referring back to again, whereas the internet, you don't know whether the site you looked at four or five years ago is still going to be there, is still going to have the same information, whereas books you can always count on.
>
> (User 6)

> [the internet] is great, but it doesn't seem to help me much, hasn't helped me, but that's probably my fault 'cause I haven't used the system properly, but perhaps that's because it's not meeting my actual – the way I want to find information.
>
> (User 3)

These comments point to the wider social, cultural and organizational issues associated with internet use, in particular the need for human intermediaries, for alternatives such as books, and to the need for information literacy-type skills so that it can be used effectively to reach self-defined goals. In a study of the use of the internet in reference, Ross and Nilsen (2000) found that reference staff regarded the internet as an external resource that users could search independently, at home or on the library's public access workstations, but not as a fully fledged reference tool for which reference librarians had a responsibility to help users search and evaluate. Next, we explore how library staff in our study used the internet in the context of a health information enquiry.

Most staff had only basic training in use of computers and the internet, in most cases the European Computer Deriving Licence (ECDL). Training and support for using the internet in the context of health information enquiries were nonexistent. Library staff who worked on the enquiry desk were asked about their knowledge of online health resources and related skills and knowledge: 'Online health information, I'm not an expert. I've never had training. I'm aware of the NHS Direct and there must be other websites, but then are they trustworthy?' (Staff Member 2).

Given this rather low level of experience and training in online health information retrieval, it is perhaps not surprising that, when going online in the course of a heath enquiry, most staff relied on the government-sponsored website NHS Direct (NHSD) and/or the Google search engine. NHSD was preferred by most because it was seen as a safe option in an otherwise 'dangerous' world of online health information:

> I mean, it's not that I won't use it but I'm very, very careful to say to people to try and find an official sounding website. Things like the NHS websites and the Social Services websites and things like that.
>
> (Staff Member 16)

We found a surprising lack of confidence among library staff in using the internet to support health enquiries. Some of their comments seem to suggest fairly low levels of information literacy, particularly in the area of information appraisal, judging its quality and relevance to the case before them. Here we may surmise that their lack of confidence may be contributing to their assertions that appraisal was beyond their expertise, assertions to which we now turn.

Staff members were asked about their practices in relation to advice, interpretation and appraisal of information. As the library literature (discussed earlier) suggests, these are difficult and yet crucial issues for library services to consider, particularly in the context of their roles in supporting active citizenship. Information and advice were seen as distinctly different. A library manager stated: 'I think that we're all quite clear that we're not here to give advice as such, we're here to help people find what they want, but we don't want to get involved in actually giving advice' (Manager 1); a staff member was equally clear: 'Our role is to guide people to where to find the information; we can't give medical advice' (Staff Member 4). However, as the next account suggests, the boundary between information and advice is not always clear in practice and is one that staff often had to struggle to maintain:

> I don't tend to commit myself to that, because we don't give advice. We do only give information. And yes, sometimes people say, 'What do you think that means?' And I suppose you sort of give your opinion on something like that. Maybe that's not quite giving advice. But no, I mean, I try not to, because I don't feel I'm qualified to.
>
> (Staff Member 10)

The subject of appraisal raised similar concerns. Staff members were asked about whether they were ever asked to help users judge the quality of the information. There was a little more ambiguity here than with the information versus advice issue. One in particular felt very strongly that library staff should not engage in 'information appraisal':

> No, because you can't do that. You can never say 'good' and 'bad' because Thalidomide was considered good by doctors ... and the fact that for years dentists gave everybody mercury fillings, and said it was perfectly all right and now suddenly it isn't, you know you really don't know what's right.
>
> (Staff Member 16)

This comment is interesting because it highlights again the need to examine the relationship between information sources and content. Even though she may not wish to comment on the content of information found in particular sources, like many of her colleagues, she is nevertheless engaged in processes of judgement, about reputable sources in particular.

The experiences of library staff illustrate well the complexities of supporting health enquiries from members of the public, especially where there is no clear diagnosis or where doctors have given only minimal guidance on what information to look for. Library staff are clear that they 'only give information', even though in practice they are being asked to get involved in diagnosis, interpretation and appraisal of information and in giving advice.

What are the implications of staff's practices in mediating health information for users' experience, and how does this fit with notions of empowerment as found in e-health discourse versus the production of a more 'active citizen' identity or subject position? A key issue here is how far staff were willing and able to support the development of a critical e-literacy among users.

We asked staff about their perceptions of users' needs in relation to judging the quality of health information online. Like many of her colleagues, this member of staff felt that users were unable to judge the quality of health information found online:

> Not really able to be quite honest. If somebody's in the medical profession ... they would be that, otherwise, the general public, I don't think they are very well able because they have difficulty even to do the simplest search on Google anyway. To get that far and that's evaluating, I think a lot of people believe what they see, really. It's all on the internet and if it is on the internet it must be OK, and they don't understand about responsibility for information ... they'll believe anything – not from me but from the internet.
>
> (Staff Member 2)

Asked whether she thought the library service had a responsibility for supporting users in this area, she seemed hesitant:

> Our responsibility is to match a personal enquiry, what they're trying to find out and to give them the best available information, but we are so pressurized and rushed up there there's very little time, you have to work so quickly in a very short period of time, um, it's very, very difficult answering questions online. I suppose we have a responsibility, but I don't know if it's an official responsibility, it's kind of a moral responsibility to find the information for somebody and make sure it's trustworthy, but when you're that rushed and other people are in the queue, jumping up and down and the phones are ringing it's very hard. We end up getting out of our time really.
>
> (Staff Member 2)

Staff in the library we studied adopted two main strategies in working on a health enquiry: they tended to look up something for the user and simply hand over the book, internet print-out or photocopied sheet, or point the user to the shelves or the internet where they could look for themselves. There was little sense that members of library staff were able to get involved in transferring any of their own information retrieval and literacy skills to users:

> We tend not to sit with them and actually help them. We do sessions for people,[3] but that is about learning for the internet rather than helping them find information.
>
> (Staff Member 15)

This same member of staff agreed that libraries could, in theory, play a more active role in facilitating user engagement with the internet for health information seeking, but that this was not current practice. She suggested that, in her library at least, staff were polarized between leaving users to search alone or providing them with the information, neither of which facilitates the type of critical engagement with online health information necessary for active e-health citizenship.

In the absence of time, political will and, quite possibly, the skills necessary to support the development of critical engagement with health information resources, staff tended to fall back on the notion of 'gateways' by which they meant portals such as NHS Direct, or sites sponsored by 'official' organizations, such as the Muscular Dystrophy Society. However, as one staff member said in reference to 'non-official' or 'alternative' sources, 'There's no reason why they shouldn't have it, they could turn out to be the right people in the end but you have gateways for official [sources]' (Staff Member 16).

Conclusion

In this chapter we have argued that in order to understand the extent and nature of the public library's role as health information intermediary, or info(r)mediary, we need to look at the wider socio-political context within which the debate has arisen. In this context, we have argued, it is helpful to think about the library's role in the context of e-health discourse, which we have defined as a combination of both the new public health (NPH) and e-society discourses. In the NPH discourse, public libraries are positioned as key providers of consumer health information, providing access to health information in the local community and helping to empower users. At the same time, the provision of free internet access in public libraries, linked to notions of 'digital citizenship' (in initiatives such as the UK's 'People's Network'), positions public libraries as key agents of change in the so-called e-society. We have suggested that there are clear imperatives and 'duties' associated with e-health discourse, as well as subject positions for both library staff and users to occupy.

In our analysis of data collected in a study of health information seeking in a public library, we found both widespread take-up of, as well as some resistance to, the understandings, imperatives and subject positions/identities offered in e-health discourse. On the whole, library staff promoted the idea of the library as provider of consumer health information with a key role to play in the support for the newly responsible and informed health consumer. Similarly, many users were happy to identify with the informed health consumer identity readily available to them in e-health discourse. However, tensions and contradictions were found in the data which has enabled us to argue that there are signs of resistance to this discourse and the meanings and practices that it implies. This was particularly the case in relation to the very particular sociotechnical configuration found in the library we studied, where the self-service model of delivery was deemed less than satisfactory by many staff and by some users, who wanted or needed access to a human intermediary. Many members of staff felt that health enquires were fundamentally different from other enquiries, often requiring more time and sensitivity on the part of library staff.

More importantly perhaps, although staff presented themselves as intermediaries (in the sense of neutral 'go-betweens' linking people with appropriate and relevant resources) in a manner consistent with the practice literature of professional librarianship as described by Bella et al. (this volume), the data suggest that their role may be far from straightforward in this regard. As we discussed, library staff members' response to the 'dangers' of the internet in the context of health information is either to encourage users to search alone or to access, or advise users to access, only a very limited number of government-sponsored or approved websites. Two issues arise here that relate to Foucault's knowledge–power relation discussed in the introduction. First, leaving relatively inexperienced users alone to search the internet may result in their accessing what Lash (2002) has termed 'informational knowledge' where the roots/contexts of the knowledge production are lost, making the kind of critical engagement with information necessary for active citizenship very difficult. E-health information accessed via the web may actually inhibit rather than support the emergence and sustainability of 'health-e citizens'. It becomes impossible to assess the validity of information if its knowledge-based roots are obscured. The use of Google as a key search strategy by library staff and users may well be contributing to the establishment of a new phenomenon: the health information 'take-away', consumed but never fully digested.

The other strategy used by staff to overcome the perceived danger of the internet as a health information resource presents a different set of problems. In promoting only government-approved sites and official 'gateways', themselves comprising only 'expert knowledges', they are presenting the information found there as 'safe', as 'neutral' information, fit for consumption by the public. In this practice, the library staff (and, indeed, the library service as a whole) might be understood as not simply 'connecting' people to the 'relevant sources', but as 'mediating' that interaction in the sense of being involved in an act of 'translation' (Silverstone, 1999: 21), a process that is itself constitutive of knowledge (Williams, 1977: 99–100). This practice can be understood as quite paternalistic and undermining of the possibility of a more active engagement with health information necessary for e-health citizenship.

It is a basic premise of much work in science and technology studies that technologies are not always appropriate solutions to social problems and that wherever technologies appear to be imposed as solutions, we should ask what the original problem actually was. This is clearly a useful way of refocusing on the social and examining the limitations of technical solutions to social problems. For example, might e-health solutions be being imposed on people whose priorities and needs might be better met through different sociotechnical configurations? In the context of the public library, expertise in information literacy would seem to be a crucial part of the sociotechnical configuration needed to support active e-health citizenship, but our research suggests that the particular sociotechnical configuration at place in the public library we studied, with the self-service delivery model at its centre, militated against this particular learning.

In the context of thinking about the role of public libraries here, it is not difficult to see how they could play an important part in encouraging a more proactive engagement with the internet among library users. However, in the library we studied, the way in which the internet was positioned both physically (in a separate room with human support for technical but not information literacy) and symbolically (as part of the self-service ethos of the organization) worked against this particular development.

This chapter has raised issues that came to light through the analysis of data drawn from the study of health information seeking in just one library in one city in one country. Thus, we do not claim that the practices we observed are in any sense generalizable. Nor do we suggest that there is necessarily anything wrong about the ways in which this particular service chooses to deliver its health information agenda. Rather, we suggest that, precisely because this library service is not alone in being positioned as a key agent of change in the e-health discourse, the challenges it faces are worthy of reflection and may be of interest to libraries and library services elsewhere. Thus, we intend our discussion of this one case not to close down debate about the public library services' role in supporting the emergence of e-health (or health-e) citizenship but rather to open it up and encourage greater reflection, in the academic literature, in policy circles and in the services themselves.

Notes

1. The study on which this chapter is based was undertaken between January and August 2006 and explored health information seeking in the context of a large city centre public library in the southeast of England. More than 200 library users who visited the library in search of health information completed a questionnaire about their use of health information resources, including the internet, as well as their experiences in the library. In addition, in-depth interviews were held with 15 library users, 16 members of staff and three managers about how they experienced either making (users) or supporting (staff and managers) health information enquiries. The study was undertaken in partnership with the city's library service, although the arguments put forward in this chapter are those of the authors alone. The study was funded by the Social Sciences and Humanities Research Council of Canada as part of the Action for Health programme (see Acknowledgements).

2. The term 'e-society' is often used synonymously with the term 'information society'. Many international, interdisciplinary conferences and workshops have been held to examine the technological, social, organizational and cultural contours of the information or e-society. In the UK, a five-year, £6.5 million ESRC funding programme has produced detailed and sustained critiques of the 'e-society': see www.york.ac.uk/res/e-society/.

3. There was just one set of 'sessions' running at the time of our study. This was a 'Silver Surfers' session aimed at introducing the internet to the over-fifties. It was the only internet training that was core-funded. Other initiatives would have to be project-funded.

4

To Filter or Not to Filter: Legal and Ethical Aspects of Librarians' Use of Internet Filtering Techniques

Elaine Gibson and Jan Sutherland

From virtually anywhere that an electronic signal can be received, a world of information is at our fingertips and hours of research can be reduced to minutes just by keying a few well-chosen words into a web portal. It is difficult to control the quantity of the information received, and the quality can range from wholly accurate and reliable to grossly misleading and even dangerous. In our homes it is up to us to judge what is useful and safe and what is not. When public institutions like libraries provide patrons with internet access, it may behove them to exercise some control over what sites are accessible as the potential for harm exists – particularly for those searching for health information.

Internet content filters are designed to control the information accessed by computer users. As such, filters mediate information through their effects on the ability of users to acquire information. Insofar as libraries choose to use filters or not, or to use them in some departments and not others, library administrators are implicated in this process of mediation, albeit tangentially, as their actions may restrict, transform or bias the information available to users. Regulation in the 'circuit of culture' is exemplified by the legal framework for decisions about the use and implementation of filters (du Gay et al., 1997; see also Wyatt, Harris and Wathen, this volume). Moreover, it is clear that the legal framework has implications for the production and consumption of information, a point to which we return in the conclusion.

In this chapter, we examine through a legal and ethical lens the use of content control filters which aim to screen out inappropriate websites. Our focus is the public library environment, as these institutions have been the focus of efforts to control access to information. We first briefly review the place of the library in information dissemination. Following that, we look at the prevalence of health information on the internet. We then discuss the nature of filters and their effects on searches for health information. The legal regimes of four countries – Canada, the United States, the United Kingdom and Australia – are surveyed with respect to internet censorship and filters. Next we examine library responses to the pressure to resort to filters. We conclude with a brief discussion of the ethical issues raised by filters.

Libraries as regulators of information

Libraries strive to be repositories of good information available to the public. Despite increasing economic pressures, public libraries are viewed as a public good worthy of support in that they serve many important functions (see also Henwood et al., this volume). In *Dividends: The Value of the Public Libraries in Canada*, Finch and Warner (1997) found that, among other benefits, libraries provide information cost-effectively, support the local economy, encourage life-long learning and promote Canadian culture. A Florida study found that public support of libraries both encouraged democratic participation and was good for the economy in that every dollar invested in the public library system returned over 6 dollars (Griffiths et al., 2004).

Libraries are also viewed as a social good. Public libraries play a role in fostering social meanings, encouraging participation in democratic governance and transmitting cultural ideals. According to Curley and Broderick:

> Traditionally, public libraries are seen as being civilizing agencies within society. This view sees the library as attempting to provide people with information and knowledge which it is hoped will lead to wisdom and understanding.... Another purpose of the library in a democratic society might be called the civic aim. The public library offers citizens of a democracy the means by which they might become informed and intelligent citizens.
>
> (1985: 2–3)

The American Library Association (ALA) produced a list of *12 Ways Libraries are Good for the Country* (2000) which expresses some of the social value of libraries. Essentially, libraries preserve the past, encourage creativity, provide family enjoyment and somewhat level the playing field between rich and poor by providing resources to the less well-off free of charge.

Libraries both represent themselves and are represented as playing a vital role in the intellectual, cultural and democratic development of individuals and the community. In fulfilling this role, libraries play a dual function: on the one hand, they provide access to information that may be inaccessible to many people, and, on the other, they play a regulatory role in the dissemination of information. By choosing certain materials over others and by restricting some materials to certain groups, libraries play a part in regulating what is validated as information worth knowing and by whom.

The representation of the library as an educational and democratizing force presses into and reinforces its regulatory role. This is particularly apparent in collections development. The very nature of collections development means adjudicating the worth of materials, but libraries are also bastions of intellectual freedom and are thus loath to engage in censorship. The representation of libraries as a social good means that the public for the most part trusts them to make correct judgements about materials. It is assumed that materials are adopted by libraries because they are good materials. Libraries, in a sense, act as gatekeepers of what is worthy knowledge and as brokers of what is essential to our cultural, political and social life.

In keeping with their role as an information resource, libraries have embraced the internet. Yet the internet threatens a loss of control over the information available, as information professionals cannot verify the information accessible via the worldwide web. The prevalence of pornography and other objectionable materials on the internet has forced libraries to grapple with easy access to inappropriate information and to consider installing filters. Internet filters[1] are clearly a technological intermediary standing between users of computers and the world of information accessible on the web. Filters play a regulatory role in information seeking in at least three respects. Most obviously, filters regulate the kind of information that is permitted to come to the information seeker. Second, by denying some kinds of information and permitting others, filters both reflect and reinforce cultural norms regarding what is acceptable and worthwhile. Finally, filters are often themselves the response to legal pressure to control information; the law in some jurisdictions mandates their use. In this sense, filters are the technological tools of the social and legal impulse to protect people, above all children, from information that may be harmful or upsetting.

Filters are an especially problematic response to the issue of easy access to inappropriate materials in libraries. Users of filtered terminals and even the libraries themselves are often unaware of what sites are blocked.

This means that filters are fundamentally different from normal collection decisions in that collections personnel make decisions based on generally accepted criteria.[2] Filters essentially pre-screen information before an information specialist can assess its appropriateness. Internet filters automate part of the function of librarians and interfere with their identities as trained professionals skilled in regulating the public's access to good information.

The internet and health information

The internet is a significant and increasing source of health information. Eysenbach and Kohler state:

> Based on our analysis we estimate that approximately 4.5 per cent of all searches on the web might be health-related. Although health-related queries constitute a relatively small fraction of web-searches, the absolute numbers are still impressive: Google reports 150 million searches per day on all regional partner sites combined, which means that about 6.75 million health-related searches *per day* in Google alone are being conducted. In comparison, in 1996 NLM reported 7 million searches in the MEDLARS (Medline) system *per year*.
>
> (2003: 229)

A study by the Pew Internet and Family Project (2005) reported that eight out of ten internet users had searched for health information online. Rideout (2001) examined access to online health information by teenagers and found that among the 90 per cent of 15–24-year-olds who have ever gone online, 75 per cent had used the internet to find health-related information, with approximately 45 per cent looking up information about pregnancy, birth control, sexually transmitted infections and HIV/AIDS. Among those who access online health information, 39 per cent reported they had changed their behaviour because of information garnered and 69 per cent spoke with friends about the information they had found. Another study by Rideout (2005) found that 53 per cent of adults aged 50–64 had searched for online health information.

There are a host of issues regarding the accuracy and quality of health information available in an unregulated environment like the internet. Among these are concerns that people will find inaccurate information online and follow it to their detriment. Quack cures and misinformation are abundant and it is often difficult to know what information is sound. Another concern, and the one most responsible for the internet filter industry, is the availability of pornography. Without some kind of content filtering, the most innocuous search is bound to include pornography 'hits', as pornography site owners often use wide-ranging metatags to attract audiences. Health-related searches are susceptible to drawing pornographic sites because both concern the human body. One means to reduce the possibility of retrieving pornographic sites is to use filters designed to screen them out.

Internet filtering technologies

The worldwide web is estimated to include over 11.5 billion pages (Gulli and Signorini, 2005). Stark (2006) estimates that 1 per cent of websites that Google and MSN index are pornographic and that 6 per cent of queries retrieve a sexually explicit web page. Even 1 per cent of the vast internet universe means that pornography is prevalent. The desire to exert control over what sites are available is understandable, particularly where access to the internet is being offered to the general public, and all the more so where minors are accessing information.

There are three main means of filtering: content filtering, exclusion lists and inclusion lists.

Content filtering occurs when sites are blocked because they contain certain forbidden key words (breast, sex, gay) or suspect graphical data such as a large proportion of flesh-coloured images. Content filtering can also work in conjunction with a rating system known as Platform for Internet Content Selection (PICS). In this instance, webpage developers rate their system according to the PICS standard and insert this rating as metadata. Filters then block out pages rated as unsuitable. Exclusion lists work by blocking access to specific web addresses or to domain names that are 'blacklisted'. Exclusion lists are generated either manually by humans designating sites as unacceptable or by automated computer searches which generate a list of inappropriate sites. Inclusion lists block all sites except those that are expressly permitted (white-listed). Inclusion lists are used infrequently as they are the most restrictive; they appear to be most often used in repressive political regimes and in the children's section of some public libraries.

Filters may be implemented at three levels. First, they may be deployed at the client level where the program is downloaded to the individual computer. The purchase of a program to screen out sites available to children on a home computer is an example of client-level implementation. Filters are also included on web browser programs and the user can set the sensitivity level to suit their tastes. Second, a filter may be implemented at the server level so that all computers on the server network are filtered. Third, it can be implemented at the internet service provider (ISP) level where the ISP filters information going to recipients of the service.

In terms of levels of consumer control over what gets filtered, filters often have restrictiveness settings where one can determine what kind of information is blocked. Internet Explorer, for example, has an option called 'content advisor' where users can block sex, violence, alcohol use and, to use their terminology, content that sets a bad example for children. However, as discussed below, using these broad categories to block information does not convey precisely the nature of the sites blocked because the decision regarding content is generally not controlled by the software user but by the vendor. It is often extremely difficult, if not impossible, for users to easily determine what websites are being filtered, since the list of what is censored is considered proprietary information and generally not disclosed.[3] Thus, while users can sometimes adjust the sensitivity of the filter, they cannot necessarily know what is being blocked.

Filtering something as vast and dispersed as the internet cannot be accomplished with perfection. Two main difficulties with filtering technologies are over- and under-blocking. Under-blocking occurs when sites that ought to be blocked are not and inappropriate materials are easily accessed. Over-blocking occurs when legitimate sites are blocked because the filter erroneously classifies them as inappropriate (Kongshem, 1998).[4] Thus, a site dealing with breast cancer may get blocked because the word 'breast' also occurs in pornographic sites.[5] Sites may be placed on the blacklist because they are wrongly classified as inappropriate or are intentionally blocked by the vendor. *TIME Magazine*, for example, was blocked by CYBERsitter after its online site posted a tool which allowed readers to type in a word and discover which sites were blocked by CYBERsitter (*Blocking Software FAQ*, n.d.). Similarly, progressive organizations like the National Organization of Women have been blocked (Meeks and McCullagh, 1996).[6]

In his expert report for a legal challenge by the American Civil Liberties Union to the federal Children's Online Protection Act (1998),[7] Stark (2006) analysed over- and under-blocking by various internet filters. He reported that '8.8 per cent to 60.2 per cent of sexually explicit websites in the Google and MSN indexes [were] not blocked'. With respect to over-blocking, Stark found that 'of the clean websites catalogued by Google or MSN ... 0.4 per cent to 23.6 per cent [were] blocked by filters'. He concluded:

> Generally, if a filter blocks more of the sexually explicit websites, it will block more of the clean websites. To take an extreme example, a parent could block all sexually explicit websites by turning off the computer. The filter that blocked all but 8.8 per cent of the sexually explicit websites in the Google and MSN indexes also blocked over 22 per cent of the clean websites.

Filtering and health information

Given the frequency of over-blocking, it is reasonable to assume that health information is highly subject to it. It is an unfortunate fact that, because much of the health information that people seek involves a body part or parts, health information and pornography employ a similar vocabulary. In addition, many parents want to control the information their children access about sex, and filter vendors particularly focus on screening out discussions of sexuality and gender.

The most comprehensive study to date on filters blocking access to health information was conducted in 2002 by the Kaiser Family Foundation (Rideout et al., 2002). The study tested the six most commonly used internet filters against 3,053 health websites and 516 pornographic sites. The researchers varied the restrictiveness of the filters from least through intermediate to most restrictive. Interestingly, given the purpose of the filters, the researchers found that varying the restrictiveness of the settings did not significantly alter the number of pornographic sites blocked. At the least restrictive settings, 'the filtering products block an average of 87 per cent of all pornographic sites; at the intermediate level, an average of 90 per cent of porn sites are blocked, and at the most restrictive configuration, 91 per cent of porn sites are blocked' (Rideout et al., 2002: 7). On the other hand, varying the restrictiveness did affect the amount of health information that was blocked. They found that:

> When set at the *least restrictive* level of blocking ('pornography only'), filters block an average of 1.4 per cent of all health sites; this figure is the average across all six of the institutional filters tested, and across all of the various health topics studied.
>
> When set at the *intermediate* level of blocking, filters block an average of 5 per cent of all health sites.

When set at the *most restrictive* configuration, 24 per cent of all non-pornographic health sites are blocked.

(Rideout et al., 2002: 6)

The study also found that sexual health sites were more likely to be blocked. When using the terms *condoms, safe sex* and *gay*, one in ten sites were blocked at the least restrictive setting. At the intermediate level, *condom* blocked 27 per cent of the health sites, *safe sex* blocked 20 per cent and *gay* blocked 24 per cent of appropriate health sites.[8]

In another study, Su et al. (2004) tested internet filters against searches using terms related to women's health in three countries. Using Google configured to three countries (the United States, China and Germany), they searched for terms with Google's filters off and on. They found that:

> The proportion of relevant women's health web sites that were blocked was quite high. For the Chinese language web sites originated (*sic*) in China, 72.6 per cent of the blocked web sites were relevant. For the German language web sites originated (*sic*) in Germany, nearly half (49.4 per cent) were relevant. For the US English web sites originated (*sic*) in the US, 95 per cent were relevant. We concluded that people might unknowingly miss potentially important health information due to information filtering.
>
> (Su et al., 2004: 1313)

Interestingly, the filters used in this study were not stand-alone products sold by vendors but simply the filters used with standard web browsers. Many people are unaware that Google comes with a SafeSearch filter that it is set to moderate by default (www.google. ca/intl/en/help/customize.html#safe). If Google's filter is set to a restrictive level and is combined with a filter sold by a vendor, the amount of over-blocking could be substantial.

Over-blocking can interfere with health information seeking. But it is also the case that there is a significant amount of pornographic, offensive and harmful materials on the internet. For people accessing information on their home computers, minimizing risk is their own responsibility, but in libraries, where computer access is supplied as a public good, those who deliver the service must try to balance allowing 'good' information in and screening out 'bad' information. Libraries have had to deal with the question of whether there should be filters placed on public access computer terminals to block access to pornographic and dangerous sites. In the next section we examine the legal regime governing this question in Canada, the US, the UK and Australia.

Filtering and the legal regime

The law is, of course, the exemplar of regulation. However, the legal systems of nations have been challenged by the internet due to difficulties in policing information originating in other jurisdictions. The difficulty in enforcing laws regarding internet content has provided an opportunity for resource exploitation by posting obscenity, hate speech, dangerous information and a host of other inappropriate materials. In responding to the 'Wild West' environment of the internet, the legal regimes of Canada, the US, UK and Australia face the difficult task of attempting to preserve freedoms of speech and expression while policing harmful content. In this section we examine various responses to the issue of filtering and internet censorship.

Protection of speech and expression

The four countries we examine all place a high value on preserving a space for the free exchange of ideas. Both Canada and the US have explicit constitutional protection for the exchange of ideas, whereas in the UK and Australia the protections are more by way of convention.

The Canadian *Charter of Rights and Freedoms* explicitly guarantees the freedoms of thought, belief, opinion and expression. Courts have interpreted expression broadly to include any non-violent expression, the aim of which is to convey meaning. It applies to political speech, commercial speech and even child pornography. However, freedom of expression is not an unfettered right in Canada. The *Charter* rights of Canadians can be curtailed if such limitation can be justified in a free and democratic society. Thus, hate speech and child pornography, while forms of expression, are limited because in various cases courts have found limits on those forms of expression to be reasonable.

In the US, there is a strong constitutional right to free speech as protected in the First Amendment. Laws and regulations that attempt to censor ideas are often found unconstitutional. Thus whereas certain forms of hate speech are prohibited in Canada, they are constitutionally protected in the US. Attempts at the federal level to censor the content of materials on the internet have been found to be unconstitutional. In the case of *American Civil Liberties Union v. Reno* (1997), the Supreme Court agreed with the ACLU that provisions in the Communications Decency

Act, which made it a felony to use the internet to send or display indecent material that could be seen by a minor, violated the freedom of speech protection of the First Amendment.

In the UK, there is no constitution and thus no constitutional right to access to information or freedom of speech. However, the Human Rights Act 1998 incorporated the EU Convention on Human Rights, which therefore became part of UK domestic law. Article 10 of the Convention guarantees a right to freedom of expression.

In Australia there is no explicit constitutional protection for freedom of expression. In *Australian Capital Television Pty Ltd v. Commonwealth* (1992), the High Court found that there was an implied right to freedom of political speech. This would not provide a constitutional protection for indecent materials under Australian law. Nevertheless, the law appears to be highly liberal with respect to such materials.

Legislation and internet censorship

In each of the four countries, obscene materials and child pornography are illegal and subject to the criminal law. Therefore all of these countries attempt to regulate internet content in some manner. Nevertheless, the degree of censorship and the means by which it is accomplished vary. Our discussion focuses on ways in which the laws affect the issue of internet filters.

In Canada, there are currently no federal or provincial laws that require the use of filters on computers in institutions, such as public libraries, which receive government funds. ISPs are also not required by law to offer filters, though most companies do. There are some forms of internet censorship in the form of provisions of the *Criminal Code* (1985) dealing with hate speech, child pornography and obscenity.

In the US some forms of expression, including obscenity, are not protected under the First Amendment as they are considered a danger to society. The US does have a more robust notion of freedom of speech than the other countries under review; nevertheless, in 2002 legislators passed the Child Internet Protection Act (CIPA). CIPA requires libraries that receive universal service discounts or funds under the Library Technology Services Act to use internet filters on all computers to prevent minors (defined as those under the age of 17) from accessing materials that are obscene, pornographic or harmful to them. If libraries do not comply, they face the loss of federal funding. Many libraries and library organizations have expressed their unwillingness to follow CIPA, viewing it as a form of censorship. However, the threatened loss of funding provides a strong incentive in favour of compliance.

The constitutionality of CIPA was challenged in *United States v. American Library Association* (2003). The American Library Association (ALA) argued that CIPA was unconstitutional because it requires libraries to violate the First Amendment by using filters to censor a substantial amount of protected speech. In a 6:3 decision, the Court found that the use of filters was analogous to collection decisions of libraries: libraries are entitled to make decisions about what they will keep in their collections without being caught up in First Amendment issues and, by extension, the use of filters is not unconstitutional.[9] In our view, internet filters are not analogous to collections decisions. Certainly, collection decisions result in the exclusion of some materials but the decisions are made on principled grounds and can be challenged. Filters screen information before anyone can make a principled determination on the suitability of the materials. Thus, while librarians are tasked with regulating information, with internet filters the locus of control is shifted to the vendor and not to those who have expertise in information management.

The Court found that CIPA did not violate the First Amendment partly because librarians can easily and quickly unblock filtered material or disable the filtering program at the request of adults and therefore do not truly block access to constitutionally protected materials. However, the wording of the legislation is vague in this regard. CIPA states that the library 'may disable the technology protection measure concerned, during use by an adult, to enable access for bona fide research or other lawful purpose'. As Jaeger et al. note:

> CIPA does not require that libraries disable filters for adult patrons, only stating that they may disable them for cases of 'bona fide research or other lawful purposes.' These vague terms are not defined in the language of CIPA and are clearly open to interpretation for librarians when they try to determine what constitutes 'bona fide research or other lawful purposes'. This leaves librarians in a possible position of feeling they have to question adult patrons about why they want the filters turned off and to make value judgments about the patron's rationale.
>
> (2005: 107–8)

The outcome of the CIPA challenge means that librarians may be required to directly regulate a patron's access to information. The issue of whether libraries must remove filters for adult use is now the subject of litigation. In November 2006, ACLU filed suit against the Northern Central Regional Library District in Washington State (American Civil

Liberties Union, 2006). The suit charges that the libraries refused to unblock computers for adults who requested that the filters be removed for legitimate research purposes. The District's internet policy apparently did not provide for unblocking computers at the request of adults (Cole, 2006). Interestingly, two of the four plaintiffs were engaging in health-related research.

The UK has traditionally had fairly robust censorship laws; in the past many works of literature have been declared obscene and subject to censorship. In light of this, it is interesting that the internet has generally not been censored.

Neither Australian internet users nor ISPs are required to use filters, though ISPs are required under the National Filtering Scheme to offer filters to their subscribers (Coonan, 2006). As part of this scheme, the National Library of Australia will be required to place filters on its public computers, with staff permitted to remove them for adult users. The filters will be offered to all other libraries in Australia but, according to the Communications Minister, funding for libraries will not be tied to whether they implement them (Pash, 2006).

Civil law

In addition to the regulatory framework outlined above, another factor that may incline library professionals to use filters is to avoid suits by patrons offended by content found on public access computers or by parents whose children have accessed inappropriate sites on the internet.

In the pre-CIPA American case of *Kathleen R. v. City of Livermore* (2001), a mother sued a library because her teenage son was downloading pornography from its computers. Among other grounds, Kathleen R. cited a violation of her son's constitutional right to substantive due process by the library's failure to protect her son's emotional and psychological health. Kathleen R. argued that libraries represent themselves as safe places for children, yet their open-access internet policy allows children to view obscene and pornographic materials, thereby placing them at risk. In essence, Kathleen R's argument was that by assuming and promulgating an identity as a suitable regulator of information, libraries place children in harm's way. The Court dismissed the complaint, holding that failure to prevent access to pornography was not the same thing as a positive policy to provide minors with pornographic materials. Therefore, the policy of the library did not violate the boy's constitutional right to substantive due process.

Since CIPA does not penalize libraries for not using filters but merely withdraws funding, an American library's decision not to use filters does not appear to open the library up to civil liability, at least in the circumstances of this case. We have not uncovered a case similar to *Kathleen R. v. Livermore* in any of the Commonwealth countries. Moreover, on similar facts, it is highly unlikely that a case would succeed.[10]

Employment law

Filters are offered primarily to protect patrons from viewing inappropriate content, but another factor that may incline a library to consider installing a filter is to protect staff. Employers have an obligation to ensure that they provide a workplace free from harassment, and pornography has been found to be a factor in the creation of a 'poisoned work environment'. The employer's obligation to provide a harassment-free workplace extends beyond employees to include customers.[11]

In 2001 in Minnesota, employees at the Minneapolis Public Library filed a complaint with the Equal Employment Opportunity Commission (EEOC) stating that the open access internet policy at their workplace repeatedly exposed them to explicit sexual materials and sexual activity online. The workers complained to the management, but management did not take action. The only internet policy in place concerned time-limits on the computers. Management did not assist the librarians when they attempted to enforce time limits on the offending patrons, and it was only after three years of taking their concerns to management that the employees made the complaint (Adamson, 2002). The EEOC found in favour of the complainants.

Provided libraries have in place and enforce acceptable use policies, it is unlikely that an employment law complaint would be successful. The trier of fact would have to balance the right of the employee to have a workplace free of sexually explicit materials against the right of the public to access materials not actually prohibited by law.

Other than in the US, governments have tended to avoid directly forcing public libraries to install filters. The effort to regulate the content of the internet in Canada, the UK and Australia has been focused at the content provider and internet service provider levels.

Library guidelines

It is clear that many legal and social complexities arise from the confrontation between inappropriate materials on the internet and attempts to regulate the internet. As ardent supporters of the free exchange of ideas and as an institution that, historically, has made worthwhile materials available to the public, libraries have found themselves in a difficult position with respect to internet filters. We now examine the library communities' response to the issue of filtering.

Canada

The Canadian Library Association (CLA) attempts to establish a balance between upholding intellectual freedom and acknowledging the risks that can result from unfettered access to the internet. Their Statement on Internet Access (Canadian Library Association, 2000) speaks about both the responsibility to educate the public about intellectual freedom and to safeguard the relationship of trust between children and libraries. In their background to the Statement on Internet Access, Archibald et al. (n.d.) summarize the kinds of legal opinions libraries have received:

> The legal opinions offered to individual library boards and at CLA Conferences are very similar. They consider the provision of Internet service in the context of the Canadian Criminal Code and the Charter of Rights and Freedoms. In summary, the opinions advise that:

- Public libraries in Canada face some risk of liability as Internet access providers, resulting from Criminal Code provisions dealing with obscenity and child pornography.
- Public libraries are likely subject to the Charter of Rights and Freedoms, which protects freedom of expression subject to reasonable limits.
- Public libraries can minimize their liability by exercising due diligence to prevent illegal behaviour, and ensuring that they are not wilfully blind to illegal behaviour.
- Due diligence includes a wide range of measures, appropriate to the extent and nature of an entity's activities, to prevent and correct violations of the law.

This document acknowledges that there are differences *vis-à-vis* the children's section of the library. Archibald et al. quote a legal opinion regarding filtering in libraries: 'Filtering of computer terminals used primarily by children is legally permissible but is not legally required as a component of due diligence.' Archibald et al. maintain, however, that while filters respond to community concerns regarding children viewing pornography, the best approach is parental guidance in teaching children how to properly use the internet. Finally, Archibald et al. note that use of filters in the children's section does not mean that terminals used by adults should be subject to filters as well.

The internet use policy of the public library in Halifax, Nova Scotia appears to have struck a balance in accordance with the guidelines suggested by the CLA:

> The Library does not control the information accessed through the Internet and assumes responsibility only for the information provided on its own home pages. The Library is not responsible for the site content of links or secondary links from its home pages.
>
> The Internet and its resources may contain material of a controversial or mature nature. The Library neither censors access to materials nor protects users from information they find offensive.
>
> The Library is a public place used by people of diverse background and ages. There are sites on the Internet inappropriate for viewing in a public setting. Library staff reserve the right to end Internet sessions when such material is displayed. Users of Internet services are bound by the same rules as outlined in the library's Public Use of Library Facilities Policy.
>
> In keeping with the public library's role in providing age-appropriate materials for children, workstations designated for children/families will be filtered.
>
> (Halifax Public Library, n.d.)

This appears to be the approach of most libraries in Canada.

United States

The American Library Association has been at the forefront of efforts to resist internet censorship. Their position on filtering is expressed thus:

> The American Library Association (ALA) does not endorse using Internet filters in libraries, because they block access to information that is legal and useful. Filters are known to block a wide range of sites, including the FBI, eBay, Planned Parenthood, The Bible and others with information many people find helpful for school, work, health and other needs.
>
> The ALA also is concerned that the use of filters may give parents a false sense their children are protected when this is not the case. Filters are not effective in blocking all 'objectionable' material, and they do not protect against pedophiles and other interactive aspects of the Internet.
>
> (American Library Association, 2007)

The ALA recommends that libraries institute internet guidelines including requiring a guardian's signature for children to use the internet rather than relying on filters.

As discussed above, the CIPA requires libraries in receipt of federal funding to use filters on all terminals to prevent children from accessing inappropriate materials. Penalties for failing to comply with the filtering requirement are financial. A study of approximately 50 libraries conducted by the Center for Democracy and Technology and the ALA found that a large majority now use filters, 'and most of the filtering is motivated by CIPA requirements. ... Only 11 per cent of the libraries that filter confine their filters to the children's section. 64 per cent will disable the filter upon request, but fewer than 20 per cent will disable the filter for minors as well as adults' (Heins et al., 2006: 5).

United Kingdom

The UK Library Association has a strong statement about the right of access to information which declaims against the general use of filters in library computers. The policy states:

> The Library Association does not endorse the use of filtering software in libraries. The use of such software is inconsistent with the commitment or duty of a library or information service to provide all publicly available information in which its users claim legitimate interest. Access to information should not be restricted except as required by law.
>
> (Library Association, 1998)

The Guidance Notes attached to the policy continue:

> Currently there is no obligation under UK or European law for library and information services to use filtering, blocking or rating technologies. Existing legislation proscribes the publication or distribution of obscene material and child pornography. These laws apply to the Internet and thus provide protection for libraries and their users.
>
> (Library Association, 2000)

The Guidance Notes also mention the possibility of liability attaching to the use of filtering programs:

> The use of filtering software may create an implied contract with library users that they will not be exposed to illegal or harmful material

when using the Internet. In particular parents may believe that their children will not be able to access such material in a library. Such implied contracts cannot be fulfilled due to the technical limitations of the software and the fact that the decisions about what to restrict are in effect assigned to a third party. Library and information services may be legally liable under these circumstances

Libraries in the UK have responded in various ways. Manchester library has a computer policy which states:

> To minimize access to inappropriate material (websites that fall under any of the following categories: adult/sexually explicit; chat; criminal skills; hacking; hate; personals and dating; remote proxies; violence/offensive; weapons) we block certain websites and chat rooms using filtering software. This software, however, may not always prevent access to such material. If you find a website that has been inappropriately blocked you may request that the site be made available, or if you find a website which you believe is unsuitable you may request that it be blocked. In either case a Library Review team will consider your request and respond within five working days.
>
> (Manchester City Council, 2006)

An obvious problem is that it is difficult to identify sites that are inappropriately blocked if one is unaware of the site precisely because it has been blocked. The library in Ealing does not appear to use filters. They offer free internet to all adults and to those aged between 11 and 18 who have the signed consent of a parent or guardian. Those under the age of 11 may only use the internet with adult supervision (Ealing Library Service, n.d.).

Australia

The Australian Library and Information Association (ALIA) is also opposed to the use of filters. Their policy is:

> Libraries and information services support the right of all users to unhindered access to information of their choice regardless of format. Access to electronic information resources should not be restricted except as required by law and this basic right should not be eroded in the development of regulatory measures for online information.
>
> (Australian Library and Information Association, 2002)

Rather than filters, the ALIA promotes internet literacy:

> Libraries and information services proactively promote and facilitate responsible access to quality networked information for all their users, including children and young people. They enable library users to learn to use the internet and electronic information efficiently and effectively.
>
> (Australian Library and Information Association, 2002)

In response to the National Filtering Scheme, the ALIA (2006) states that it 'does not recommend the use of internet filtering technology in public libraries. Filtering has been shown to vary in its effectiveness, blocking some sites with useful and legal information, while not fully protecting children and others from illegal, objectionable or offensive material'.

Use of filters varies across libraries in Australia.[12] The ALIA conducted a survey of internet access in 2007. They found that 39 per cent of responding libraries reported using internet filters. The survey also noted that, while complaints about inappropriate content had gone down, they also received complaints about the filters (Australian Library and Information Association, 2007).

Ethical considerations

Our final section highlights some of the ethical issues that arise in the context of filtering. We look particularly at the effects of filters on the traditional role of librarians and the ways in which filters both undermine and enhance autonomy.

As discussed above, while selection decisions are necessary, such decisions are to be made on principled grounds to ensure that libraries meet their public obligations. The public trusts librarians to choose materials based not on prejudicial or biased considerations, but on what materials seem to convey worthwhile information. This task was undoubtedly easier when information was primarily print-based. Given the costs associated with printing and the vetting processes of publishers, most materials in print had some redeeming qualities. Selection choices were made by professionals or by reliance on digests compiled by professionals.

It is not surprising that the issue of filters in libraries has generated much discussion among information professionals. Nor is it surprising that libraries have responded in the variety of ways they have. Filters bring to the fore the conflict between the right of individuals to access a wide range of information and an acknowledgement of the unsavoury side of the free flow of information. The classic liberal view of the free flow of information as an unmitigated good has run into the unregulated environment that is the internet. The internet has done away with the editor, publisher and expert and, while much of what is available is valuable, anybody with access to a computer, an internet connection and a modicum of design skill can produce sites containing information that is fallacious, vicious, ridiculous or wrongheaded.

In the normal course of materials selection, libraries can be called to account for actions that are tantamount to censorship because it is possible to find out what viewpoints are consistently rejected from collections. With internet filters, vendors rather than libraries are responsible for the censorship. Libraries are required to provide the tools of censorship without controlling what gets screened out. Librarians are in a difficult position. They must determine how to use information-restricting technology that has usurped their historical role in guiding patrons to greater knowledge and self-discovery while being aware that this technology is no substitute for their expertise.

At an abstract level, important values are engaged in the filtering issue. Autonomy is one of the key values of Western society. Autonomy requires self-governance and the ability to act without coercion or interference from others (Dworkin, 1989). As autonomous agents, we have the right to live our lives as we see fit, so long as we do not infringe on the autonomy of others. Access to information is an essential condition of autonomy in that without a reasonable degree of knowledge, one cannot come to thoughtful and independent conclusions regarding issues. Libraries, then, can play an autonomy-enhancing role in society.

Filters affect autonomy insofar as they are a form of censorship infringing on freedom of thought and the free flow of ideas. This censorship strikes at both the development of the autonomous person and the exercise of autonomy by individuals. Filters smack of paternalism because they stand between individuals and the information others deem they ought not to see.

As we are encouraged to undertake more of the responsibility for educating ourselves about our health, filters play at least two roles. First, they prevent people from being confronted by images and text they may not be seeking. Health-related searches generate hits on pornographic sites and, by blocking these sites, the technology is assisting searchers to meet their own needs. However, over-blocking may result in individuals failing to find the information they are looking for. The same search, then, can result in something that is both autonomy-enhancing and a barrier to autonomy.

Furthermore, much of what is on the internet is neither valuable nor autonomy-enhancing. One of the major criticisms of pornography, the material most subject to filtering, is that it creates conditions that deny women in particular their full humanity. Perhaps limiting access to that kind of material is not such a harm to people. In this sense, the censorship afforded by filters is autonomy-enhancing as it removes from contemplation what many would argue degrades members of society and reinforces ideologies that keep women from fully participating in public life. This may be the position that a more relational concept of autonomy would direct, as we are forced to look beyond the narrow bounds of the individual, their ideas and their actions and acknowledge that we are engaged in a context rich with social meanings that can be channelled or challenged.

The use of filters in the children's sections of libraries may well be ethically defensible. However, their use in adult areas is ethically questionable. Moreover, abdicating responsibility to filter vendors for selecting what materials should be screened out may be surrendering too much control over the shaping of public discourse, particularly when such products over-block. As well, this surrender of control fails to encourage the development of information literacy, which ultimately can affect participation in public life.

Finally, it is worth noting that the legal and social pressures to regulate internet content have primarily dealt with pornography and hate speech. Little has been done to regulate commercial speech, and thus there has been no concerted effort on the part of legislators to intercede in the problems caused by 'quackery' and biased health information on the internet. Filter vendors do not attempt to screen out factually bad information. The fact that filters censor sexual materials over materials that may prove more directly harmful, such as the promise of 'quack' cures or the potential for bias in commercially sponsored health information, deserves greater focus and attention in future.

Conclusion

Two important conclusions emerge from this chapter. The first is that filters are an important, albeit often invisible, form of mediation, as demonstrated by Balka and Butt (this volume). It is clear that internet filters affect health-related searches on the internet. The hope is that as the technology improves, the proportion of good information that is screened out will be reduced. There are solid reasons, including legal requirements and social pressures, why librarians might want to use filters, especially in the children's section. There are also solid reasons why libraries might want to forgo their use, given the mandate of libraries to serve the public. Decisions about the use of filters are not clear cut given the dangers inherent in an unregulated internet.

The second conclusion concerns the role of regulation. Understanding the legal framework in which filters are regulated and used provides insight into the production and consumption of information, the other elements of the circuit of culture (du Gay et al., 1997). The use of filters constrains the apparently boundless choices offered by the internet, so that information producers may not always be able reach their intended audiences. Consumers – in this case library users – are also affected not only by the filters themselves but also by the legal framework regulating their use. Within public libraries, a decision about the use of filters is not in itself sufficient. Where filters are utilized, they should only be part of the library's internet strategy, which should also include the development of internet use policies and measures to increase computer literacy. Patrons will thus be assisted to access accurate, reliable and inoffensive information. An important element of computer literacy, for both library staff and library users, is an awareness of the possible presence of filters and what this may mean for the nature of the information that becomes visible during online searching. This is especially the case with respect to health information.

Notes

1. Content control software also goes by the names 'censorware' and 'web filters'. In this chapter, we use the term 'filter' as, to our minds, it is the most accurate description of the technology, since the control over content is by means of filters.
2. See, for example, the Halifax Public Library's *Collection Development Policy* (1997).
3. The company which produces CYBERsitter threatened to sue an anti-filtering website called Peacefire after Peacefire provided a program which would decode the list of sites blocked by CYBERsitter. The lawsuit was never pursued (*CSDecode*, n.d.)
4. Kongshem includes the following quote: ' "Using a computer that had Surfwatch installed on it, I was able to download information on how to build a bomb, how to contact a satanic cult, how to sabotage various systems within a building, read up on neo-Nazi propaganda, and learn how to commit crimes

using cellular telephones", says Bill Lowenburg, a librarian and technology trainer in the Stroudsburg (Pa.) Area School District. "On the other hand, I was not able to access the English Server at Carnegie Mellon University, because it apparently had 'objectionable' content on it".'

5. For a comprehensive report on what gets blocked by filters, see Heins et al. (2006).

6. A recent criticism of filters is that they do not block advertising and marketing aimed at children. Indeed, in some cases those who produce filters profit from the advertising (see Freschette, 2005).

7. This Act would have required all commercial distributors of material harmful to a minor to restrict minors from accessing the site. ACLU obtained an injunction prohibiting the enforcement of the Act and argued the case before a federal district court. In *American Civil Liberties Union v. Gonzales* (2007) the Court issued a permanent injunction against Children's Online Protection Act finding the legislation was an unconstitutional infringement on the First and Fifth Amendments and was overbroad and vague.

8. The report does not state the levels of blocking at the most restrictive setting.

9. The Court failed to acknowledge that commercial vendors were making decisions as to what to block rather than professionals who have a commitment to presenting divergent points of view on topics of interest to citizens.

10. For an analysis of the tort liability of librarians for injury caused by online content in Canada, see Sutherland and Gibson (in press).

11. See United States Equal Employment Opportunity Commission (2007) or Canadian Human Rights Commission (2006).

12. For example, the State Library of Western Australia uses filters on its computers (State Library of Western Australia, 2005) whereas the State Library of Queensland does not (State Library of Queensland, 2006).

5
Invisible Logic: The Role of Software as an Information Intermediary in Health Care

Ellen Balka and Arsalan Butt

Driven by citizen demand and supported by government, the area of e-health covers a wide range of socio-technical innovations in health service delivery and organization, ranging from electronic patient records and hospital administrative computer systems to end-user consumption of online health information. Information technology applications in the health sector have made it possible to consolidate numerous and varied sources of information. For example, patients and their families can use the internet to search for information about health and illness online. With the emergence of online health information, the internet was often viewed as an optimal way to disseminate health information because it offers privacy, immediacy, a wide variety of information and a variety of perspectives (Bischoff and Kelley, 1999). As the internet has expanded to address the demand for medical information on health-related topics (McLeod, 1998), optimism about internet health information seeking has cooled, and although emphasis on internet-based health information as a means to empowerment continues (Masi et al., 2003), many recent studies which have explored the dynamics surrounding online health information consumption present a more nuanced view (Henwood et al., 2003; Pitts, 2004).

Health information websites have been supported by government health policy documents in many countries, suggesting the belief among policy-makers that availability of online health information will lead to the emergence of more informed patients, better able to assess the risks and benefits of different treatments for themselves. For example, a Health Canada planning document identified as a priority the provision of 'relevant, credible and timely health information to the public to empower individuals to manage their own health through a Canadian Health Network and self-care and telecare services' (Health Canada,

2000: 79). Consumer health information is often seen by policy-makers and health information consumers as central to patient empowerment and consumer/patient involvement in health decision-making. However, the equation of the consumption of health information by patients/consumers with patient health and empowerment has not escaped critical scrutiny (Henwood et al., 2003). Although the rhetoric of empowerment surrounding the introduction of internet-based health information has been strong, many questions remain about the equation of internet health information seeking and empowerment. It is often assumed that health information seekers go online, find information that addresses their concerns and then use that information in an empowering way. 'Empowerment' in the context of online health information seeking is often portrayed as an uncomplicated relationship between an individual, a computer and an information source, with little attention paid to the complicating circumstances of the seeker, the knowledge base or motivation of the information producer, or the mediating roles that computer hardware and software may play in the process of information exchange (cf. Figures 1.1 and 1.2 above). In this chapter we consider the role that software plays in health information consumption processes in general, and in making online health information either accessible or inaccessible to health information consumers in particular. Our aim is to highlight the role that software plays as an information intermediary in online health information seeking.

Research reported here was undertaken as part of a project[1] that had as one of its goals to 'explore the use of the internet as a means of gaining access to health information, and specifically, to determine what roles information intermediaries (people and/or hardware and software who help information seekers find the information they need) fill when those around them seek health information via computers' (Balka, 2003). The term 'intermediary' describes varied configurations of humans and machines which may help or hinder people as they search for health information. Information and communication technologies (ICTs) can be conceptualized as one type of intermediary in that they provide access to information that would otherwise not be accessible, and present particular contextual circumstances that may help or hinder access, comprehension and usefulness of information. As Wyatt et al. (this volume) suggest in identifying ICTs as an intermediary, the mediation of information also occurs in relation to the underlying technological infrastructure of hardware and software. Software and hardware play a role in mediating the information retrieved by online health information seekers – before they actually see it. In processes which constitute online health information seeking – undertaken in varied contexts ranging from end-user consumption of health information in the context of health promotion or self-care, to the use of data about the health system by researchers, operational staff or policy-makers – computer hardware and software can be thought of as infrastructure.

As infrastructure, technology is often rendered invisible if it is working well (Bowker and Star, 1999). As Star (1995) points out, computer systems simplify and make choices about voice, politics and knowledge that are often invisible. Such decisions embody power in their ability to encode some parts of human life while excluding others. These decisions often have consequences that are not immediately apparent. For instance, information seekers may be unaware of the role that hardware and software may play in ordering the information they retrieve or the ways that particular hardware and software configurations can render some kinds of information visible and other kinds of invisible.

In this chapter, we discuss the intermediary role of computer software in health information retrieval. Drawing on a detailed case study that addressed lower than anticipated use of BC HealthGuide (BCHG) OnLine, a health information website funded by British Columbia's provincial government, the means through which software may structure the flow of information received by end-users is explored and discussed in relation to du Gay et al.'s (1997) circuit of culture, and in particular the concepts of regulation, consumption and production. Findings from our research are used to illustrate how computer systems can affect the visibility of health information. We conclude by suggesting that while information systems, in their varied forms, may increase the amount of information that people see, a limited understanding of the ways that this information is shaped by underlying software may hinder health information users from achieving their desired goals. While in some cases increased accessibility of health information may be altering relationships between health information providers and users (e.g. many doctors report that patients now come to clinics armed with printouts from online health websites, ready to challenge the notion that 'doctor knows best'), it appears that existing practices are leaving power hierarchies of technical experts and information users in many senses unchanged. Information users remain unaware of the significant role that software plays as an information intermediary, and many health information seekers now unknowingly abdicate the role of information intermediary to the search engines they use to access online health information.

Consumption of online health information

BCHG OnLine has been utilized to a lesser degree than is perceived as desirable by its funder, the provincial Ministry of Health in British Columbia. Although 55 per cent of British Columbian households reported, in 2003, at least one member who regularly used the internet for health information seeking (Statistics Canada, 2005; Veenhof, Clermont, and Sciadas, 2005), use of the BCHG OnLine website was significantly lower than this benchmark. Despite improvements to the BCHG website in 2005, only one in four British Columbians were aware of it, a finding consistent since January 2004 (Balka and Butt, 2006). A survey undertaken by the BCHG through its website indicated that only 27 per cent of British Columbians were aware of the HealthFiles feature (online health fact sheets about a single topic, which are formatted to be downloaded and given to patients) and that search engines were the most frequently used resource by health consumers (65.5 per cent) prior to their use of the BCHG website (Prosser, 2006). Although utilization of online resources does not in itself result in the empowerment of health information seekers, if there is any possibility for empowerment to occur as a result of consumption of online health information, being able to access online health information will be a prerequisite. It is our view that the notion that consumption of online health information will lead to empowerment is quite simplistic and problematic, and because of the prevalence of this view in policy and patient discourses, it warrants closer examination. Here we shed light on why such views are problematic through investigation of what has been described as a problem (the lower than desired rates of use of the BCHG OnLine) by the BC Ministry of Health which provides funding for BCHG OnLine. Examining the lower than desired use of the BCHG OnLine website provides a mechanism through which various aspects of software as an information intermediary can be explored.

Regulating health information: software as information intermediary

Several possible reasons for lower than anticipated use of the BCHG website[2] were identified. The main one was that online health information seekers did not easily find the BCHG website when searching. The second possible explanation was that potential users may have been finding the site and not returning to it if they were unable to meet their health information needs on the site.[3] In order to probe these possibilities we pursued two strategies. First, we conducted searches to see if we could 'find' the BCHG website;[4] we then recruited participants from three groups (parents with young children at home, seniors and youth)[5] to conduct searches in a controlled setting to see if, when they searched online for health information, their search strategies located the BCHG website. We subsequently interviewed the participants individually and as part of a focus group to learn more about their views of the BCHG website.

From our observations, and the interview and focus group data, we concluded that the visibility of the BCHG website could be improved through technical optimization strategies. More important for the purposes of the present discussion, both our own and end-users' search activities yielded insights into the role of software as an information intermediary and about processes of regulation which come to bear on the distribution, production and consumption of health information (du Gay et al., 1997).

Introna and Nissenbaum (2000: 171) suggest that 'web page providers seeking recognition from search engines for their Web pages must focus on two key tasks: (a) being indexed and (b) achieving a ranking in the top 10–20 search results displayed'. In our systematic searches of the BCHG website,[4] it appeared on the first page of search results only 20 times out of its total 50 appearances in 94 searches. This can have strong implications for the frequency of its use and its components because users do not always look beyond the first page of external search engine results, a finding supported by data collected during observations of users conducted as part of this study. If people cannot find the site, they will not be able to use it. Users may also develop a 'bad impression' of the BCHG website if the site appears in a list of returned results but the link leads to information which is not on topic. Hence, it is significant that in search results 40 of 50 appearances of the website were irrelevant to the search queries. Too many inappropriate results can deter users from viewing a website. Use of common colloquial terms (which most of the participants in the focus groups used in their searches) produced ten irrelevant results on the external search engines, and 28 of 94 queries on the internal search engine also produced irrelevant results. Although optimized keywords to match content of pages indexed can be employed to address this issue, the often well-guarded secrets of the intricacies of search engine algorithms make it difficult to make websites visible.

Introna and Nissenbaum (2000) provide a detailed overview of the strategies that search engine designers and operators use and the choices they make about what is included and what excluded from their databases, choices and decisions that, more often than not, are commercial secrets and hence invisible to end-users who search for online information. These choices are 'embedded in human-interpreted decision criteria, in crawl heuristics, and in ranking algorithms' (Introna and Nissenbaum, 2000: 175). Introna and Nissenbaum suggest that all search engines return only a portion of the relevant information that is online; they argue that 'the partiality of any search attempt (even if we assume a competent searcher) will magnify the problem [of bias] in the context of search engines' (2000: 177). This is particularly problematic because users may not be aware of the inherent partiality of search engine results.

As the example above indicates, software, however invisible, matters. The decision to use one search engine rather than another has an impact on which results are returned in response to a search query, and hence can effectively determine what information a health information seeker sees. In this way, software in general and search engines in particular can serve as intermediaries which regulate access to online content. Some content (in this example, non-Canadian content) is rendered more visible than other content. Clearly, search engine design is only one mechanism of several that together determine what content is visible to health information seekers. Other important ingredients include users' search behaviours, technical variables (such as how content is 'tagged' and hence how it is located by search engines) and broader legal or contractual issues which may dictate one approach to making content visible (content tagging) over another. During the planning stages of our study, we interviewed two staff members who worked at the BC NurseLine (a telephone line accessible 24 hours a day, seven days a week) who relied on call centre software developed by the same company that provides content for BCHG OnLine. In those interviews, several examples emerged of instances where the combination of user search behaviours and how content was tagged resulted in situations in which BCHG OnLine users followed unsuccessful web-based searches with telephone calls to the BC NurseLine.

Carrying out systematic searches as described above allowed us to assess the relative visibility of the BCHG website when using various search engines, but told us little about health information seekers' search behaviours, which clearly can – and do – influence access to content. Our interest in better understanding how health information seekers went about their search tasks led us to devise a multi-method strategy for which we recruited three groups of health information seekers (parents, seniors and youth). They came to a community centre where we gave them health scenarios (again, based on the 'top five' queries received for their group by the BCHG NurseLine call centre) and asked them to search for information related to the scenarios as they would at home, insofar as that was possible.[6] Ideally, we would have observed people searching for health information of their choice in the setting where they normally engage in search activities, as such *in situ* observation yields a more accurate picture of actual behaviour. However, because online health information seeking occurs in varied locations and at unpredictable times of the day, we had to devise another method to learn about health information seekers' search habits and strategies, which led us to the quasi-experiment outlined here.

Google.ca was the most frequently used search engine (the only search engine used by youth) among the eleven health information seekers we observed.[7] The BCHG website did not appear in search results for any of the youth participants. When google.ca or yahoo.ca (which has a similar feature that allows users to filter for only Canadian content) were used, participants never used the software option that filtered out non-Canadian content. This was particularly interesting given comments we heard during the focus groups about the desire to be able to locate more information about local health services online. This desire did not lead health information seekers to select an option in their search engines that would filter for more locally relevant content.

From observing health information seekers while they conducted searches, we learned that participants' normal search strategies did not lead them to the BCHG website at all. By associating keywords with content, search engines can better categorize a website. In addition to content that is already written into a web page, keywords can be added through use of meta-tags. The current BCHG OnLine home page and a large number of sub-pages do not contain any heading, strong or emphasis tags. Appropriate tags could be used to allow search engine spiders[8] to better understand the website's contents, and various other search engine optimization strategies could be utilized to improve the visibility of the BCHG OnLine website.[9]

Information is readily available about how to improve the visibility of websites in relation to search engines, which raises questions about why the BCHG OnLine website remains so invisible to search engines, and consequently potential users. It would be tempting to dismiss the poor visibility of the BCHG OnLine website as what Nettleton and Burrows (2003) have identified as a 'supply-side barrier', an impediment 'associated with providers, such as poor management' (Nettleton and Burrows, 2003: 171), marketing or other provider issues such as staffing. Other supply-side barriers include an inability to develop sites of interest to target populations, or an inability to engage desired users. Our data suggest that while some supply-side barriers might be at play (for example, youth participants took offence that data about their age cohort had to be accessed through a link that applied to anyone who was aged four or older – a feature that did not entice them to come back to the site), the relative invisibility of the website might reflect other issues.

In a discussion which situates health information seeking within the broader context of risk culture, Nettleton and Burrows (2003) suggest that Giddens' (2002) theory of reflexive modernization (a process of modernization that is characteristic of risk society whereby progress is achieved through reorganization and reform) 'has been transformed from being a sociological *description* to becoming something more akin to a political *prescription* for the restructuring of the welfare state' (Nettleton and Burrows, 2003: 169). In other words, ideas about reorganization and reform of the health system have moved from being mere ideas about how to achieve progress, to prescriptions to be followed about achieving progress through certain types of reform – in this case, consumption of online health information rather than interaction with health professionals. Government enthusiasm for such websites should then be understood in part as politically prescribed reform, designed to serve the interests of the welfare state as much as the interests of the individual.

Nettleton and Burrows go on to argue that such views presume 'that individuals are rational actors who consciously, carefully and reflexively seek out information to improve their lot' (2003: 169). Our observations of online health information seeking behaviour suggest something other than careful, conscious actors who reflectively seek information. Drawing on Lash's (2002) work, Nettleton and Burrows suggest that

> reflexivity in this sense is less about reflecting and thinking and is more to do with 'reflex'; it is the act of engaging with (technological) medium that communicates the message or information ... the act or 'reflex' of sourcing information becomes inseparable from the act of assessing and responding to it.
>
> (2003: 175)

The apparent incongruity of health information seekers indicating that they desire health information that has a higher degree of local relevance than the information they retrieve, while at the same time failing to constrain their searches to information housed only on Canadian websites suggests that health information seekers may well be guided by reflex rather than reflexivity in their online searches.

The intersection of health information production, consumption and regulation

The BCHG OnLine website content is provided by a US company which operates as an incorporated non-profit organization, a designation which in the US can be obtained for organizations dedicated to education. Although a non-profit, the vendor offers a range of products for sale to health plan and benefit providers, health care providers, government and policy-makers, and health information consumers. The vendor's product line includes a database (which serves as the basis of the BCHG OnLine website and BCHG NurseLine) and a handbook, which has 30 million copies in print. Although the primary market for their products is the US, the products have been localized, or adapted, for Canadian use.[10] We initially became aware of localization processes through our research partnership with the BCHG. The research questions we pursued above did not require that we delve to the extent that we have here into issues related to localization. While preparing this chapter we conducted additional background research about the vendor and localization, which we draw on in this section.

Localization has included alteration so that content meets Canadian medical standards, Canadian prevention and treatment guidelines, uses Canadian brand names for medications and Canadian (rather than American) spelling (for example, colour rather than color). Localization of the material also addresses cultural factors. The vendor's website indicates that 'Aboriginal peoples may be mentioned as a risk category in certain diseases and conditions' (Healthwise, 2002). Investigation of the BCHG OnLine website determined that diabetes was one such condition. Using the search phrase 'Who is affected by type 2 diabetes?' in both the US and Canadian versions of the database revealed that being Aboriginal was indicated as a risk factor for diabetes in the Canadian but not in the US version. In the US version, the following phrase appears: 'type 2 diabetes is more common in African Americans, Hispanics, Asian Americans, and Pacific Islanders than in whites'. In contrast, in the Canadian version, the following phrase appears: 'type 2 diabetes is more common in people of Aboriginal, African, Hispanic, South Asian, and Asian descent'. It is not known why being of Aboriginal origin is considered a risk factor for diabetes in Canada but not in the US. Other differences in ethnic groups referred to in the above statements reflect, among other things, differences in the ethnic composition of the US and Canada.

Although the vendor's website indicates that localization has also included the addition as resources of Canadian organizations such as the

Canadian Heart and Stroke Foundation, in some instances references to Canadian organizations were lacking in the BCHG content. For example, content about a neurological disorder that typically occurs in conjunction with severe immune system compromise, including AIDS, identified several AIDS-related organizations including a gay men's health crisis line as resources, all of which were in the US. There is a vibrant gay community in British Columbia and a high degree of acceptance for homosexual people in Canada (reflected in the legalization of gay marriage), yet none of the many Canadian organizations offering similar services were listed on the BCHG website. The vendor's claims about localization appear to be overstated.

Our interview with the two staff members who worked with the BC NurseLine indicated the limitations of content localization and challenges associated with the tagging and organization of online content that affected NurseLine staff when they used the vendor's software while answering calls. For example, one interviewee pointed out that Nurse-Line received calls about street drugs with some frequency and that callers often indicated that they had attempted to locate information online prior to calling. Referring to the BCHG OnLine site, the staff member indicated that information about street drugs and rape was not easily located on the BC HealthGuide website. While the Nurse-Line staff could memorize the location of such information, potential BCHG OnLine users were not necessarily aware that the information could be accessed via another route. To complicate things, the information was only accessible if proper names (e.g. marijuana) were used, rather than colloquial expressions (e.g. pot). The staff member who conveyed this information suggested that the difficulties in locating such information in the database were indicative of differences between the US (where there is a 'war on drugs') and Canada (where there are more liberal views about the use of marijuana). Content developed in the US reflects attitudes and social mores there. Although some information about illegal drugs can be found on the BCHG website, it is limited.

The organization of information and the way it is tagged (labelled for subsequent retrieval by a search engine) within the BCHG website also renders some topics less visible. In the example above, although some information about illicit drug use does exist on the BCHG website, much of it is found under links titled 'Teen Alcohol and Drug Abuse' and 'Alcohol and Drug Problems', which may not be the first places a teenager would be inclined to look for information about smoking marijuana. Similarly, although the BCHG website contains information about rape, there is no obvious link to that information. As one of the NurseLine staff members pointed out, 'They call in and don't say "I've been raped" – they have a story. There is no rape site or websites.' Another problem is that the terminology that potential BCHG information consumers use differs from the BCHG content. One staff member commented that:

> [S]ome of that information is not in the language that those popula-
> tions use. . . . For instance, a mom calls in to say she found a joint in
> her son's room and she has been asking what to do. I'd like to write
> in joint [in the search field of the knowledge base] because that is all
> the mom knows it is called . . . all the street names of drugs should be
> searchable.

Another example that staff cited of content that existed online but was difficult to find related to information about genitals:

> [A]ny genital issues for women – you can go into it [the knowledge
> base] via vaginal but for men you have to put in [to the search box]
> male genital and not penis. For women you can put in specific body
> parts, but for men you have to go in through male genital. It should
> either be male genital and female genital, but most people call in with
> penis and vagina.

When the BCHG OnLine website was first launched, use of the website required health information seekers to enter their provincial health care number. This was an odd requirement, given that at that time, data captured when people called the nurse line or used the website were not used for any reason. Hence, the requirement to enter a personal health number may have been put in place as a device to restrict those from outside the province (who were not covered in the licensing agreement) from using the BCHG OnLine website. Eventually, the requirement to enter a provincial personal health number in order to access the website was dropped and replaced by a requirement to enter a provincial postal code in order to gain access to the website. Searches conducted in early 2007 while preparing this chapter indicate that this gatekeeping function has been removed.

Given that the costs of maintaining a website are the same whether or not all Canadians access the site or it is accessed only by those living in British Columbia, the only reason for access to be restricted to the site is a licensing agreement. If all Canadians could access the BCHG OnLine website rather than only those living in British Columbia, the vendor would, in effect, eliminate the Canadian market for its product. As long as the site is only accessible to residents of one province, the possibility of licensing the product for use in other provinces exists. Although recent changes to the BCHG OnLine website do not require health information seekers to enter a password or postal code to access the BC version of the database, access to online content is subject to varied restrictions in other jurisdictions. For example, some content from the database can be accessed through the US-based Group Health website, but when search results are returned, a notice above the results indicates to health information seekers that if they do not find what they want, they can 'log in to MyGroupHealth for access to most of our online services and resources, including in-depth Condition Centers on some common health conditions, the Healthy Living section, discussion groups, and other health information'.[11]

Our research indicated that the BCHG OnLine website appeared either not at all or so far down in the search results retrieved via various search engines that it remained undiscovered by potential site users. We further observed that search strategies used by the eleven health information seeking participants did not uncover the existence of the site. We therefore investigated the tagging mechanisms used on the site and came to the conclusion that much could be done to facilitate its visibility. That measures had not been taken to increase the site's visibility in search engines really only makes sense if one considers the implication of improving its visibility – the most direct consequence of which would potentially be the loss of revenues from possible sales to other Canadian provinces.

In spite of the non-profit status of the vendor, the need to generate revenues has implications for how content is made accessible to potential consumers. In the first instance, access has historically been restricted to the content through a gatekeeping function, as indicated above. In the second instance, access to the website is restricted through content-tagging mechanisms that make the site difficult to discover from search engines. One consequence of such content-tagging practices is that uptake of the site becomes more dependent than it would be otherwise on marketing and promotional efforts directed towards the target audience, which effectively externalizes the costs associated with obtaining uptake of the site to the agency that has purchased the content. Hence, the software serves as an intermediary, regulating the accessibility of content and subsequently the use of information by users. The production of the information within an environment where revenue generation from sales is important is reflected in content conventions (e.g. poor tagging), which also serve a regulatory function, at times restricting the visibility – and hence accessibility – of the site. The invisible logic of the software – search engines and tagging conventions – has played a role as information intermediary, more often than not unknown and unknowable to the information seeker and the provincial funder.

Making logic visible: other forms of software intermediation in the health sector

Our analysis of the BCHG Online website has provided a context in which we have been able to introduce the concept of software as an intermediary and to demonstrate how the combination of software (search engines) and content (how it is tagged) serve as filters and influence what health information people can see. This example illustrates only one of several ways that software functions as an information intermediary, coming to bear on what information is visible (and hence what can be known) and rendering other information invisible. Another instance in which the invisible logic of software and hardware constraints can act as an information intermediary, regulating the availability of information, relates to the assumptions that content designers make about the computing systems through which users will access content.

Closely linked to the example discussed above are issues related to hardware and software configurations of computer systems, which can effectively limit the access some users have to web-based health information. For example, websites that feature sophisticated graphics may not be accessible to anyone with a low-speed connection to the internet, and websites that use the latest programming languages may make content inaccessible to those with older computers, which are not robust enough to run newer operating systems or accommodate the latest form of content that has been incorporated into web pages. Continual development of new media forms that can be delivered via the internet (which now include videostreaming and audio content, as well as text and varied forms of graphics) fuels a need for frequent replacement of computers and effectively limits the accessibility of health information to those who are unable or unwilling to engage in nearly continual upgrading of computers.

Conclusion

In this chapter, issues related to software as an information intermediary have been outlined in relation to the consumption of online health information and use of the BCHG website. It is, however, important to realize that in virtually all e-health applications in the health sector, whether they are health information web portals, disease-based registries or electronic patient records, the software behind these applications serves as an information intermediary and the consequences of its design are hidden from most users. The assumptions and goals of system designers (e.g. the desire to generate sales of the database, which initially resulted in limited access to the BCHG OnLine website), as well as the behaviour of users (for example, not selecting the 'pages from Canada' function when searching online for local health information), come to bear on the specifics of how software regulates the flow of information, often in ways not readily apparent to users. This occurs in part because the logic of the software is hidden from view of most users, who use computer software and hardware in an environment that does not encourage people to problematize the role that infrastructures play in organizing the world (Bowker and Star, 1999). Software developers' design decisions (e.g. tagging web content so both proper and colloquial language retrieve a result in a search engine) also have an impact on information consumption. Furthermore, the profit imperative and other interests are reflected in technical decisions made at the stage that information resources are produced. As the examples here have shown, the invisible logic at the heart of software warrants attention because it plays an important role in determining what information is available to users, and in turn what they can know. Increased accessibility of health information, whether to patients and their families or health decision-makers, can only lead to empowerment if the invisible logic of software is made visible to those who rely on it to deliver information to them.

Notes

1. This work was undertaken as part of the Action for Health project (see Acknowledgements).
2. Possible explanations for low use include (i) lack of awareness due to poor marketing, or the site not being easily located online because of tagging or licensing issues; (ii) content not interesting or useful to information consumers; and (iii) content not easily accessible due to poor fit between website and user or user and designer, or poor usability.
3. This latter line of thinking was inspired in part by data that suggested that a high proportion of those who responded to a BCHG online survey were first-time visitors to the site. This has caused our research team to wonder if users visit the site, fail to find what they are looking for and subsequently do not return.

4. For the first approach, researchers entered key phrases into a range of search engines with the goal of determining where the BCHG website appeared in a list of search results. The selection of search engines was based on the existing literature that identifies search engines that are used by health information consumers (Connor, 2000; RAND Health, 2001). The comScore media Metrix ratings (Sullivan, 2006) of search engines were also used to identify the most frequently used search engines by English-speakers worldwide. The systematic searches were based on the top five topics, for each of the populations included in our study, of calls to the BC NurseLine, a telephone nurse advisory service also funded by the Ministry of Health. A total of 94 searches were conducted on five external search engines (Google.ca, MSN.ca, Ask.com, Altavista.ca and Yahoo.ca), as well as the internal search engine on the BCHG website. The BCHG website appeared 50 of 94 times, and in 20 of the 50 instances where it appeared, it was on the first page of results. When the BCHG internal website was used to search for topics known to be on that website, in only two-thirds of the searches were the results displayed relevant to the searches undertaken. We also learned that search results that include the BCHG website appear in Canadian searches (that is, .ca sites or Canada indices only) more often than global searches and that the BCHG website is better indexed on Google.ca and Yahoo.ca than it is on Altavista.ca; it did not come up at all on Ask.com. Searches on Google.ca were conducted with and without the option of 'pages from Canada' selected (by default, Google.ca searches without selecting the 'pages from Canada' option). A link for the BCHG website did not come up in the first five pages of searches done unless the 'pages from Canada' option was selected. This could be a potential obstacle to the visibility of the BCHG website, and other Canadian websites, to online users as users may not always type .ca (instead of .com) in search engines, and search engines do not always identify users' geographical location automatically.

5. In this chapter, 'seniors' refers to adults over the age of 65. 'Youth' are young adults, aged from 16 to 24. 'Parents with children at home' includes parents with children under the age of 18 living at home.

6. We also had them repeat this process from within the BCHG OnLine website. See Balka and Butt (2006) for more information about research methods.

7. Five individuals aged between 21 and 23 years (three females and two males) participated in the 'youth' focus group. All were university students who considered themselves expert internet users. Two males and one female between the ages of 38 and 45 participated in the 'parents' focus group. The 'parents' had children between the ages of 3 and 19. Male participants self-identified as expert internet users, while the female participant thought of herself as an intermediate internet user. The seniors group included two men and one woman, and were aged between 66 and 71. The female senior considered herself a novice internet user, one of the senior men identified as an advanced user and the other male self-identified as an intermediate internet user.

8. Search engine spiders are programs that browse the web in a methodical, automated manner; they create a copy of all the visited pages for later processing by a search engine that will index the downloaded pages to provide fast searches.

9. See Balka and Butt (2006) for more detailed information about the BCHG website, and Introna and Nissenbaum (2000) for an overview of tagging and other issues related to searching.

10. The localization strategy can be found at http://www.healthwise.org/p_online_cont.aspx#hwkbc. The US version can be found at: http://www.ghc.org/kbase/topic.jhtml?docId=/hw132609/hw132609.xml; and the Canadian version at: http://www.bchealthguide.org/kbase/frame/hw132/hw132609/frame.htm

11. See http://www.ghc.org/kbase/index.jhtml for US-based Good Health Guide and http://www.ghc.org/Find/searchResults.jhtml?_requestid=749099 for the notice cited here.

6
Personalized Narrative Diagnostic Imaging: Can it Mediate Patient–System Dialogue?

Peter Pennefather and West Suhanic

Much of the disease burden in North America is due to chronic illnesses that need to be managed at either an individual or a population level. People living with chronic diseases account for 75 per cent of health care expenditures in the United States (Hoffman et al., 1996). To both define and judge care outcomes and guide adaptation of the health care system to the individual and societal burden of chronic diseases, a continuous flow of diagnostic information is needed. The field of diagnostics involves the practice and science of delivering this flow of information. Recent analyses of information-ordering and use in medical practice have emphasized the fluid mutability of this information, depending on context (Moser and Law, 2006). Based on the reflexive feedback delivered by diagnostic tests during therapy, best practices and clinical guidelines are continuously adapted by health care professionals. Ideally, this dynamic and informed approach to standards also improves practice over time provided there is a record and a rationalization of the context dependent adaptations. In this chapter we explore how this process of interpretation could be influenced if diagnostic information was packaged and presented in a way that reflects not only underlying biomedical processes, but also the patient's perspectives and concerns.

A wide range of diagnostic information is interpreted visually and can be represented in a format that can be stored in an image file. Diagnostic images are ordered at critical periods in the ongoing interaction between an individual and the health care system to help guide that system in responding to that person's needs. This stream of diagnostic events and the records that they produce provide important reference points that can be used in describing the person's trajectory through the health care system. Here, we explore how a diagnostic image file, contextualized and resident within a network of electronic patient records, might act as an information intermediary between the person with the health problem and the health care system assigned to that problem. More specifically, we explore how that intermediary role can help to anchor a narrative of goals and expectations of persons receiving care within the goals and expectations of the health care system. The diagnostic test record modified in this way thus can act as an information intermediary that can enable ongoing dialogue between patient and system.

Many forms of digital diagnostic images are used to probe and document the causes of a person's disease and the state of that person's health. Diagnostic images can range from x-rays (e.g. medical diagnostic imaging) to micrographs of a clinical sample (e.g. tissue-based diagnostics). Generally, these are now captured and stored digitally. Without contextualization, the data in such files, and even the pictures generated by reading them, are not very useful. Some of these rendered images are not even pictures in the traditional sense. They are interpreted projection maps of signals detected by scanning focused energy beams through the body, such as scans generated by magnetic resonance imaging (MRIs) or computed tomographic x-ray scans (CTs). To be clinically useful, these digital files need to be interpreted with full knowledge of the rest of a patient's medical records, as well as knowledge of the instrumentation and the purpose of the diagnostic test. Image-based diagnostics is thus a branch of health informatics that includes much more than the process of recording and storing a digital image. An informatics *system* is based not only on computers but also on clinical guidelines, formal medical terminologies and information and communication technologies. It is applied to constructing a diagnostic story around an anatomically defined region of the body as well as around pathophysiological mechanisms.

Here, drawing on du Gay et al.'s (1997) circuit of culture, we explore how the regulation and production of technology are embodied in the integration of these image files within an idealized comprehensive health record system and consider how this integration might support a narrative diagnostic imaging process. By narrative diagnostic imaging, we mean an extension of the diagnostic imaging informatics system that includes recorded 'images' of patients' worldviews, and their goals for interacting with the health care system. We believe this process could enable a mediated dialogue between a patient and the health care system as it is represented by the 'circle of care' of health care professionals who are directly responsible for various components of patients' care. We examine current interactions between the production and regulation of the diagnostic imaging systems and explore how a new form of patient-mediated qualification of these images might arise through simple and feasible modifications of existing procedures used to generate, archive and share diagnostic image files.

Braman (2006: 16) has argued that tightly controlled information perceived as having a high degree of facticity can take on agency. Given the weight placed on the results of expensive medical diagnostic imaging tests, we propose that the information associated with these tests can also take on agency. We apply that term here in the sense used by Rose and Jones (2005) in developing their concept of the 'double dance of agency'. They propose that information systems can have agency, but only in the sense that the information interacts with and makes a difference to human agency. Diagnostic images can directly affect the course of treatment by their mere presence in the patient record. They influence the decisions of members of a dynamic 'circle of care' who make professional decisions regarding the person's health care, based on the medical evidence available to them. For example, CT scans and MRIs of a brain tumour are used in tandem to determine when and what form of brain surgery is needed. In some cases, discussion within the circle of care concerning the location and size of the tumour, as well as the context in which the person is living, will lead to a recommendation to *wait and see* rather than to immediately resect the tumour and thereby take on additional health risks always associated with brain surgery. Thus, diagnostic testing and the utility of diagnostic images do not end with naming (diagnosing) the disease. In many types of chronic disease it is not possible to eliminate the cause. Rather, much of chronic disease therapy is aimed at mitigation, preventing dangerous symptoms from emerging, and improving as much as possible the quality of the patient's life.

Our analysis points to opportunities to begin aggregating, annotating and tagging primary digital diagnostic images to enable them to fulfil a broader function than simply recording the primary results of isolated diagnostic events. We propose that these digital images can take on a number of other useful roles, including: 1) becoming a 'container' for related clinical and personal information relevant to interpretation of the digital image; 2) co-localizing meta-data with the original image; 3) serving as a communication bridge between the person and their care providers; 4) linking the community-of-care with information sources relevant to the person's condition and the group's information needs; and 5) providing reference milestones in a mutually developed narrative of the person's experience of his or her transit through the health care system. These enhancements would allow the image to tell the patient's story – hence the term 'narrative diagnostic imaging'.

Diagnostic events are initiated for a specific clinical purpose at a specific time and place. They therefore have the potential to serve as a guide to the clinical logic underlying the course of events recorded in patients' medical records. Diagnostic images embedded in patients' records can help to illustrate and highlight care episodes. They can anchor patient-focused narratives which chronicle health seeking experiences, promoting the concept of narrative medicine (Kay and Purves, 1997; Charon, 2001). Narrative diagnostic imaging provides a means of linking biomedicine and health care system meanings and realities to patients' cultural, social and biological meanings and realities.

Health care system trends driving a capacity for narrative diagnostic imaging

In both Europe and North America, governments are committed to establishing inter-operable electronic patient record systems before the end of 2010 to complement paper-based medical records. The goal is to catch up with most other sectors of society where electronic record-keeping and enterprise resource planning systems are becoming the norm. This push for national electronic health record (EHR) systems is being driven by the increasing complexity of medical care and the associated decrease in both the quality and safety of health of care despite ever-larger health care expenditures (Leape and Berwick, 2005; Woolf and Johnson, 2005). In parallel, there is a movement towards the establishment of patient-controlled personal electronic health record systems (PHR) that enable patients to aggregate all electronic medical information relevant to their health and then authorize access to care providers as needed (Mandl et al., 2001; William et al., 2005).

The digital nature of most diagnostic images used today means that there is no technical barrier to incorporating them into hospital-based electronic medical record systems (EMRs) and from there into EHRs and PHRs.[1] Indeed, the need to share medical records, especially medical image files, has been a major driver for such record systems (see below). This raises the possibility that the image file can be highlighted with tags and other forms of digital information relevant to patients that could assist them to present their stories within the health care system.

The individual being cared for usually has the clearest overview of their convoluted trajectory through the health care system. This is leading to more explicit engagement of patients in controlling the course of his or her treatment. Evidence points to the importance and effectiveness of patient self-management in guiding the course of treatment plans that are often poorly coordinated (Lorig et al., 1999). This evidence, in turn, is driving innovations such as the Expert Patient Program[2] in the UK (Donaldson, 2003) to assist people living with long-term illness to manage their condition and develop more control over their lives. There are also attempts to train and reimburse a subset of patients to guide others who face similar challenges. These trends reflect an increasing recognition of the need for patients to be able to recount as accurately and precisely as possible what they have experienced.

Most EMRs are now designed with the capacity to allow patients to review and identify errors in the record. This review function has been extended to EHRs and PHRs. We propose that such functionality should be extended to allow patients to enter comments about their feelings and concerns as well as specific questions about what they can expect from the course of their disease given the results of diagnostic tests. These questions and comments would need to be answered and, in principle, this could create a medium for communication between the patients and the health care system that is grounded in their progress through care plan-guided therapy. This line of communication could (again, in principle) support a rich dialogue around qualifying and personalizing the contents of these electronic records.

Next, we explore how digital files that record the results of diagnostic imaging events could be modified to serve as broader information containers to enable qualifying commentary from multiple sources to be overlaid on the primary data and displayed whenever primary data are used. These containers could also incorporate reports of patients' experience of their disease and their care at the time diagnostic images are recorded. This approach of co-localizing biomedical and personal/clinical data within the same file structure and using the same file locater to access that personal view would ensure that the health care system users' perspectives are evident in the information artefacts used by the health system to assess patients' health care needs from the system's perspective.

Biomedicine trends facilitating narrative agency roles for diagnostic images

Major trends in the practice of biomedicine are increasing the importance of the results of diagnostic tests for guiding health care decisions and documenting health care outcomes, as well as increasing the agency function of the test results themselves. Two of these trends will be considered in detail here: 1) the uses of biomarkers as more precisely definable surrogates for physical signs and symptoms traditionally used to diagnose disease progression; and 2) disease management strategies and programmes developed to capture and represent general experience with the expected course and outcomes of therapeutic best practices informed by diagnostic test results.

Biomarkers

Advances in our understanding of cellular and molecular biology, as well as new methods for monitoring biomolecularly determined cellular processes, have ushered in an age of molecular biomedicine. A molecular biomarker is a molecularly definable characteristic that can be objectively measured and evaluated as an indicator of biological, pathological or therapeutic processes. Biomarkers can provide information about: a disease or drug target (type 0); a drug or its mechanism (type 1); or a clinical outcome (type 2). Biomarker analysis can range from a simple measurement of blood glucose or cholesterol to measurement of a spectrum of endogenous metabolites that is then interpreted through the lens of sophisticated systems biology models of the *metabolome* (a description of the interaction of all bodily biochemical reactions) (Frank and Hargreaves, 2003).

The identities of diseases are being redefined in terms of biomarker surrogates for established clinical signs and symptoms (Cambrosio et al., 2006). Increasingly, recording of medical images of body regions or micrographs of clinical pathology samples are explicitly carried out with the aim of quantitatively measuring discrete and molecularly definable biomarkers. *In vitro* diagnostic tests are also emerging with little direct relation to the person with the health problem and understood instead in terms of a fundamental biomolecular process. Diagnostic images used to measure, monitor and map such biomarker surrogates within individuals or populations take on new meaning as key artefacts used in representing and understanding a person's disease within the health care system (Frank and Hargreaves, 2003). In order to balance this biomolecular conceptualization of disease, there is a need to directly link biomarker representation of disease with personalized understanding and representation of the disease experience.

Disease management

Our understanding of population health and disease mechanisms enables prediction, for specific populations, of the likely course of a disease and response to therapy in that population. This has created opportunities for instituting disease management programmes that extend beyond an immediate therapeutic intervention that happens in the hospital or the doctor's office. These programmes are often aimed at enhancing and supporting self-care efforts and often involve patient education and input by non-physicians. The concept of disease management was first developed by drug companies in the 1980s to justify consumption of drugs to reduce symptoms associated with chronic disease morbidity. In the 1990s, government and disease-based charities targeted education of patients with chronic disease. In the first decade of the twenty-first century, disease management is increasingly a health system-driven process designed to improve health care quality. This approach is becoming professionalized. Increasingly, formal definitions of disease management are emerging. According to the Disease Management Association of America,[3] disease management is a system of coordinated health care interventions and communication for populations with conditions in which patient self-care efforts are significant. A full-service disease management programme has elements of population identification, evidence-based practice, collaborative practice, patient education, process and outcomes measurement, and routine reporting loops.

Krumholz et al. (2006) provide a good overview of the concept of disease management as understood by physicians. Health care models such as *chronic health care, primary health care, case management, coordinated care, multidisciplinary care* and *interprofessional care* all have important disease management components. The targets of disease management programmes could be persons with the disease, care providers or both. Generation of diagnostic images plays a key role in many disease management services. Suitably annotated diagnostic images could therefore support decision-making within disease management programmes. They could also help in evaluating programme efficacy. In the US there are several major government-sponsored efforts to evaluate whether disease management programmes for chronic health problems can increase the value and effectiveness of Medicare expenditures in terms of cost and health care outcomes. The results of those studies are pending, but the role of disease management programmes in the health care system continues to evolve (Krumholz et al., 2006).

As with any management process that is dependent on sharing information and knowledge, doing so across boundaries is problematic (Ciborra and Andreu, 2001; Ciborra, 2002). For true adaptive and innovative management of dynamic disease process to occur, management systems must be sufficiently flexible to respect and recognize local conditions and the tacit knowledge of participants. Management guidelines should never be considered 'finished'; rather they are frameworks for mapping an ongoing learning process (Ciborra, 2002). This will be especially true when diagnostic imagery is used to guide treatment and care of people living with chronic disease. Here, the diagnostic dialogue must be adaptive, multifaceted and respectful of the contributions of all participants. It must also recognize the patient as a participant in that dialogue (Berg et al., 2005).

There is a certain amount of anti-intellectual hubris associated with the 'evidence-based-medicine' (EBM) movement (Miles et al., 2007). Academic analysis of assumptions behind the EBM movement can result in attacks on the questioner's scholarly integrity (Murray et al., 2007). Nevertheless, the promise of EBM is undeniably appealing. Improved access to processed and ordered information about best practices and validated outcomes is essential for good governance of the considerable resources invested in the health care system.

Information and communication technologies and digital diagnostic images in health care

There have been several reviews of the transformative impact of ICTs on clinical diagnostics. Medical specialties, in particular radiology and pathology, make extensive use of visually interpreted image-based diagnostic information and have been early adopters of ICTs in their practices. Most reviews of teleradiology, telepathology and telemedicine in general tend to focus on how that technology can be used to share images among distributed clinical sites and reduce duplication costs (Caramella, 1996; Lin, 1999; Weinstein et al., 2001; Moore et al., 2005). In these reviews, the image file is treated as a passive container of image data captured during a primary diagnostic event.

The image may be annotated using the DICOM (digital imaging and communications in medicine) standard format. Each DICOM file has a header containing, among other items, patient demographic information, acquisition parameters, referrer, practitioner and operator identifiers, and image dimensions. The rest of the DICOM file contains the image data. This format was jointly developed by the American College of Radiology and the National Electrical Manufacturers Association to ensure a national standard for storing and transmitting medical images. The existence of this standard has allowed development of institution-specific picture archive and communication systems (PACS) (Graham et al., 2005).

Previous authors have examined efforts now underway to allow integration of these PACS (and the images they contain) into electronic medical records (EMRs) systems (Ratib et al., 2003). Others have examined parallel efforts to incorporate the results of clinical tests, including digital image-based tests into patient-controlled PHR systems (Zhang et al., 2005). Although those reviews pay particular attention to the way in which access to the files is authorized, none has examined how the images themselves might initiate authorization for inspection and aggregate opinions as to the meaning of their contents.

Some reviews have begun to examine the significance of the increasing network accessibility of clinically significant digital diagnostic images and the adoption of the web as medium for using that resource. For example, Gortler et al. (2006) explore the potential advantages of grid technology in tissue-based diagnosis and how certain archiving and interpretive services could be distributed within a network of nodes. Gortler et al. (2006) and Ratib et al. (2003) both comment on how the emergence of open standards and an emphasis on interoperability are driving the development of applications that permit integration of information from multiple sources at multiple locations and institutions.

Web 2.0

The impact of new, internet-based collaborative knowledge evaluation services, often lumped under the rubric 'web 2.0', is beginning to be felt and discussed in medical practice (Giustini, 2006) and in the education of health care professionals. Paralleling the professional use of specialty web 2.0 services, a large number of non-professionals use Google to guide their health seeking behaviour. There is evidence that Google can be a useful diagnostic aid (Tan and Ng, 2006), however a fair degree of professional knowledge is required to interpret and evaluate documents found using popular search engines (Gardiner, 2006; and see Balka, this volume, for a discussion of search engines as a mediator).

The popularity of social networking applications such as YouTube or MySpace and image tagging software such as Flickr illustrates the potential of sharing access to digital images. The business world is already beginning to explore the significance of these trends for its activities, as are publishers of scientific literature (Hannay, 2007), raising the possibility that social networking applications will also migrate in the near future into the health care world and assist carers and patients to navigate the complex web of care services evoked even during routine interactions with the health care system.

Narrative diagnostic imaging regulation and its technological meaning

In Canada, the contents of a patient's health record, including the results of all diagnostic tests, are, in principle, owned by the patient, although care providers serve as temporary custodians of the data (ACIET, 2005). In practice that custodial role is taken seriously and access to the records is closely guarded. Ready access is restricted to a precisely defined 'circle of care' limited to certain groups and individuals who have a legal mandate to access the information. Nevertheless, this legal framework recognizes the right and need for patients to be able to gain access and comment on the content of their health records. We propose that this right to personal health information access could create opportunities to empower patients not only to make their voices heard, but to keep a record of their wishes and desires with respect to the care process.

In this chapter we have advanced the concept that digital image files containing information needed to reproduce the product of diagnostic events can become not only a technological mediator of communication between diagnostic imaging devices and health care professionals, but a mediator of communication between the subjects of diagnostic events and their circles of care. We hope that the approach can make explicit and evident the dimensions of self, discourse and power that are central to the critique of health care inspired by the writings of Foucault (Bunton and Petersen, 1997).

Concern about the regulation of non-medical use of information in the medical record has hindered implementation of electronic records systems. Patients are worried that potential employers, regulatory agencies or insurance companies may gain access to information that could stigmatize them. Health professionals, who are well aware of the risks involved in medical care, are worried that medical errors, which inevitably happen in complex care regimes, will be made more evident. Because of limited resources the fidelity of care is often compromised (Leape and Berwick, 2005; Woolf and Johnson, 2005). Compromised care does not necessarily cause harm because self-correcting interventions may rescue the situation or minimize unnecessary harm, but the best possible care is not delivered. Also, patients define medical errors much more broadly than institutional definitions of medical error (Burroughs et al., 2007). Care providers are worried about making such *patient-perceived* errors in care delivery more evident. Payers are worried about the near-term increase in costs that will accrue from making evident chronic care needs within EHRs. Indeed, EHRs have been marketed to physicians in terms of their ability to identify more problems in a way that will increase the number of procedures that can be ordered and billed for, thereby increasing physicians' income.

Although it is widely recognized that many long-term benefits could be derived from increased use of EHRs, and despite considerable financial incentives offered by governments, their use in North America has lagged behind Europe. Sidorov (2006) suggests that uptake of EHR usage is unlikely unless medical practice and attitudes are altered. The ready access and co-localization of the patient's perspective within the highly structured and objective bio-diagnostic image may help to maintain contact with the person while the health care system is busy characterizing the bio-medically conceptualized disease. This added value may be what is needed to drive changes in attitude towards EHRs.

For narrative diagnostic imaging to work, the diagnostic image needs to serve a health information intermediary ('infomediary') role between people with health care problems and the various health care providers who deal with their cases. In turn, this implies mediation of two-way transmission of information. The intermediary adapts multiple information formats in ways that make information accessible to the patient while at the same time making the patient's information needs clearer to those who provide care/information, thereby improving access to relevant information. This intermediary role requires an explicit characterization of the patient's context, experiences and identity- and health-related needs. An effective 'infomediary' also needs to be able to relay and receive information about patients and their needs. From a circuit of culture perspective (du Gay et al., 1997), we propose that narrative diagnostic imaging could be particularly useful in mediating articulation between moments of diagnostic imaging technology production and regulation. Keeping this in mind, let us examine what properties would have to be built into the image file if it were to take on that intermediary role.

First, the digital file would have to be configured in such a way as to track access to its contents and initiate procedures to present information relevant to the purpose of that access. This in turn would require functionality to interpret the purpose of file queries, negotiate access to appropriate information sources relevant to those queries and aggregate query responses in a way that improves the ability of the patient to utilize the diagnostic data embedded in the diagnostic image. Second, the file needs to be able to accommodate and contain all the additional meta-data that someone examining the diagnostic image might need in order to interpret it appropriately, as well as additional data accrued through repeated queries. Third, as mechanisms emerge whereby images with common features and tags can become associated with other similar images, the file may be able to drive a new form of social networking that links patients and their care providers with appropriate peer groups for mutual support. This latter function would be predicated on developing appropriate privacy and spam filters to ensure that the experience is mutually supportive and builds trust in the process.

We will now illustrate design features that could be developed using existing technologies in a way that creates distinct information intermediary roles for suitably enhanced diagnostic image files. What follows is a list of those design features:

1. *The file becomes a 'container' for related clinical and personal information relevant to interpretation of the diagnostic image.* The DICOM standard is an industry standard which ensures that diagnostic images are generated with additional information that allows them to be shared and communicated beyond the instrument that generated them. However, as the concept of biomarkers becomes better established, features within the image will take on additional meaning because they can be bio-referenced to other knowledge maps. There will be a need to develop a file format analogous to GeoTIFF, which allows geo-referencing of coordinates[4] within satellite images of the earth's surface to other knowledge maps containing that coordinate information. By analogy, one can imagine a BioTIFF standard that allows biomedical imagery to be linked to the anatomical coordinate structure of the body such as is represented by reference image sets generated by the visible human project.[5] The Laboratory for Collaborative Diagnostics[6] is currently developing this approach. The BioTIFF file format uses the multilayered .tif format to create a digital container capable of holding digital images and all the meta-data for those images. The meta-data can, for example, include patient ID, accessibility permissions, descriptive information about the patient, all relevant image capture information, information about the location of the diagnostic event, its purpose, and so on. Most importantly, the BioTIFF can accommodate additional meta-data and comparator diagnostic images as needed or as they become available. The .tif format can also incorporate sound and video information as well as text.

2. *The file structure simplifies subsequent use and curation of diagnostic information.* Including necessary interpretive information in the image container itself will simplify the process of managing and authorizing access, and will also protect the patient's privacy rights. It will allow the image container to be shared across multiple health care

information systems. Indeed, the image container becomes the integration mechanism. The alternative is the current scenario where each information system must contain all or part of the image container. Making sure the information systems are all updated with the latest version of the digital container is currently neither administratively nor logistically feasible.

3. *The file serves as a communication bridge between patients and their care providers.* A digital container can function as a technical integration mechanism. Because the digital container gives access to the relevant health care information through its flexible, dynamic and transportable design, it can function as a communication bridge between patients and their care providers. In this role as a social integrator, the digital container facilitates the necessary communication between all the involved parties and may result in improved care, enhanced patient safety and reduce the changes of inappropriate treatment.

4. *The file links many communities of care.* The digital container can support a lot of information that is of interest to both the container's owner and the attending health care professionals. If it is also accessible to computational agents, it opens up the potential to identifying patterns and linkages between varieties of conditions and creates opportunities for novel epidemiological studies. Indeed, the container's existence in itself can incite new types of disease surveillance not previously possible. The digital container is not only a Dawkian meme (Dawkins, 1976), but a building block that may influence the success of diagnostic programmes to prevent the spread of disease within populations and disease progression within individuals, thereby enabling programme adaptation and evolution within the information ecosystem it inhabits.

Conclusion

Diagnostic images are highly constructed and interpreted artefacts that serve to 'etch' together concepts about the physical body with political hierarchies and technical practices to construct a picture of procedures that should be invoked within the health care system to deal with disease (see Joyce, 2005). These procedures are being continuously adapted through a process of systematic recourse to the (dynamic and continuous) collective production of evidence, a process Cambrosio et al. (2006) call 'regulatory objectivity'. This is similar to the call for accommodation of reflexivity in complex ICT systems that are designed to improve the effectiveness of heath care delivery (Moser and Law, 2006; Hanseth et al., 2006). This reactive/adaptive process relies on information that is perceived to be sound and immutable. The perceived immutability of the data is driving increasing reliance on approaches such as the use of biomarkers and best practices in disease management to define disease and determine care, and leading and increasing reliance on biomolec-ular concepts. There is a need, we believe, to balance these trends towards standardization with evidence of patients' understanding of their conditions and needs. For the diagnostic information to become understandable to practitioners and caregivers in the health care system (the 'circle of care') the stream of clinical information entering a given patient's health record needs to be overlaid with personal narrative. The process of narrative diagnostic imaging described here is a preliminary attempt to design such a system.

There is no technical barrier to the introduction of a narrative diag-nostic imaging process into diagnostic imaging practices as they are now conducted. This type of imaging would embed patient-produced rep-resentations of their goals and expectations within the digital artefacts generated by diagnostic imaging procedures. Patients-authorized access to diagnostic imaging files linked to contextual and narrative informa-tion would result in new information spaces in which novel insights into health problems and treatment options could emerge within the circle of care. By applying now established principles of secondary use of health data it should be possible to adequately de-identify these records while still providing information necessary to continuously improve practice. Moreover, it would allow patients to be partners in that discovery pro-cess. However, getting this approach right requires explicit recognition and development of the infomediary role that suitably elaborated nar-rative diagnostic imaging files might play in an increasingly digital and virtual, electronic health record environment.

We propose that the diagnostic process should be considered as a form of mediated dialogue in which it is important to consider not only all of the inquirers but also the mediating artefacts, such as the digital files used to store diagnostic information and interpretations. Source and object of knowledge and meaning are bound together in a trialogical process (Paavolaa et al., 2006). This process includes interaction of both sources of information (patients and their circles of care) and meanings (diag-nostic interpretations) with the artefacts and the physical and virtual environments that embody that information (the image file in the PACS).

National health care systems are struggling to build patient record systems that can support both whole-person care and integrated care (Weiner et al., 2005). Both goals would be advanced if there was a way to customize care services reliably to meet specific, individual needs. To do this equitably, the desires and self-identified needs of patients must be represented. Narrative diagnostic imaging might be one way to achieve this goal. Beyond enabling the health care system to deliver patient-centred care that is more customized to the individual, narrative diagnostic imaging could be useful in establishing broader networks of peer-supported care and extending public health literacy. In summary, personalized narrative diagnostic imaging is feasible and could provide a new medium for patient/ health care system dialogue mediated by the diagnostic image file itself.

Notes

1. For discussion of the distinction between EMRs, EHRs and PHRs, see http://www.chip.org/research/ping.htm and http://www.ncvhs.hhs.gov/0602nhiirpt.pdf.
2. www.expertpatients.nhs.uk/
3. www.dmaa.org/definition.html
4. www.remotesensing.org/geotiff/geotiff.html
5. www.nlm.nih.gov/research/visible/visible_human.html
6. www.lcd.utoronto.ca

7
Using the Internet as a Health Intermediary: Providing Information and Services to Marginalized Sexual Communities

T. C. Sanders

Of the many information and communication technologies (ICTs) that have had an impact on public life in recent years, arguably none has been more marked in its effect than the internet. In 2005, an estimated 68 per cent of Canadians had used the internet for personal, non-work reasons in the past year (McKeown, 2006). A particularly striking trend is the popularity of the internet as a resource for health information. According to the Canadian Internet Use Survey, 58 per cent of Canadians have used the internet to search for medical or health-related informa-tion (CIUS, 2005). Similarly, a survey of seven European countries found that 71 per cent of people online have used the internet for health pur-poses (Andreassen et al., 2007). Thus, the internet is quickly becoming a popular venue for both the production and consumption of important health information. Less clear, however, is how and to what extent the information is being incorporated into people's daily lives.

The internet has vast potential to operate as an intermediary of health information between the producers of technology and information and those who consume these products.[1] Public health information can be widely disseminated free of charge to consumers with little or no cost to producers. Information about physicians and services can be sys-tematically sought and explored at consumer convenience. Information concerning sensitive issues can be located from the comfort and security of one's home. Basic patient care and medical advice can be accessed and distributed using interactive online services. DiMaggio et al. (2004) describe this information and service potential as a 'moving target' for scholars interested in analysing data exchange across multiple contexts.

As a network of networks that digitally links people and information, online technology provides an ideal site for studying the production and consumption of a broad range of medical information and services. On the one hand, online resources provide a near-limitless index of vital information that is otherwise often expensive or difficult to obtain. On the other, sceptics caution that online information is largely disorganized and often rife with half-truths and misinformation. Moreover, how online health information is distributed by providers and interpreted and implemented among users can have a dramatic impact on people's well-being. All these issues must be taken into account when attempting to ascertain the effectiveness of the internet as a health intermediary.

Men for men (M4M) websites are a form of ICT that has come under scrutiny by the health community. Since the late 1990s, M4M websites and chat rooms have become increasingly popular among gay and bisexual men seeking casual sex partners. While there is no way to accurately gauge how many sexual encounters are regularly facilitated by M4M websites, Brown et al. (2005) estimate that 35–60 per cent of men who use these sites arrange for casual sex. The websites are public and localized,[2] basic memberships are free, contain user-friendly search engines for locating other members and boast thousands of members for most metropolitan areas. In recent years, however, they have also been implicated in outbreaks of sexually transmitted infections (STIs). Not surprisingly, public health researchers concerned with the health of gay and bisexual men have developed a keen interest in these websites as a potential source for studying risky sexual behaviour among men seeking men, as well as their potential for providing safe-sex and other sexual health information. As ICTs, these websites can function as vital health intermediaries between public health professionals and, broadly speaking, a population at high risk for STIs. This marked shift could be termed a process of articulation (du Gay et al., 1997; Hall, 1997), whereby these websites have made the transition from their intended purpose as dating venues to assume a mediating role as resources of health information.

Recently, community health researchers – sometimes in collaboration with private web servers – have produced a series of online health information strategies for pilot implementation on M4M websites. At the heart of these initiatives is the use of internet technology as an affordable yet effective conduit between health information and online users. The interventions range from passive health advisory links and private online notifications e-mailed between users, to interactive public websites and chat room-based educators. These pilot projects are produced with unidirectional intent, namely to disseminate specific information that, ideally, influences or modifies the sexual behaviour of the M4M community. Examined only from this perspective, however, the relationship between ICTs and people appears purely deterministic and fixed. By contrast, I explore these online health strategies as intermediaries travelling along the ICT conduit. Seen in this light, the strategies are negotiated and sometimes contested when the goals of community researchers producing online health information and the needs of the M4M online community are at odds with one another. To this end, I adopt the 'circuit of culture' (du Gay et al., 1997; Hall, 1997) framework, which explicates the competing relations of production, consumption, identity, representation and regulation that create cultural products, broadly construed here as internet technologies. Using this theoretical perspective, the creation and use of online health interventions can be seen to operate together in a cycle of competing processes. At times, the cycle occasions unexpected outcomes that highlight the instability and creativity underlying cultural consumption, particularly where digital technologies are interactive. This chapter focuses on the use and efficacy of online health strategies marketed to M4M websites and chat rooms. I am particularly interested in the negotiation process whereby men either explore or disregard different strategies, concerns over privacy and sexual regulation, and how competing uses of online health strategies become contested through user applications.

Health science, STIs and M4M websites

M4M websites are a unique object of sociological research for exploring the relationship between ICTs and the production and use of health information. To date, however, they have registered primarily as foci of epidemiological research aimed at curbing instances of sexual risk and the spread of STIs. Public health interest in M4M websites began in the late 1990s as it became clear they were becoming increasingly popular venues in facilitating casual sexual encounters among gay and bisexual men. Specifically, health researchers noticed a correlation between this activity and recent increases in STIs. Initial studies by McFarlane et al. (2000, 2002) and Klausner et al. (2000), for example, indicated that men using the internet to arrange sex have more partners than those who do not, and that recent syphilis outbreaks were associated with men using these sites to arrange casual sex. By 2002, these findings led some health officials and researchers to liken M4M websites and chat rooms to virtual bathhouses, reporting that 'the Internet may be a setting in which to meet new sex partners and potentially transmit HIV' (Chiasson et al., 2003, 37).

Public health officials have since looked to internet service providers and website moderators to assist in combating the spread of STIs. Specifically, M4M websites have been asked to warn users of STI risks, provide static links to safer sex information and allow access to users' contact information. In some instances, service providers, such as AOL and MSN, have been threatened by public health officials with legal action for failing to comply with specific and targeted initiatives, such as pop-up windows and group e-mails, intended to supply risk assessments of specific websites (Dotinga, 2004). These events have, in turn, sparked an ethical debate about whether internet websites constitute public or private space, as well as about preserving the anonymity of individual web users. There is concern that government agencies could conceivably monitor and record online activity for the purposes of contacting users. As a result, M4M users may feel that their privacy has been violated; an accompanying concern is that closeted men may be deterred from using the websites. Such action is reminiscent of past crusades against bathhouses, which infringed the rights and social lives of gay and bisexual men, but had relatively little effect in curbing HIV transmission (Alexander, 1996; Bérubé, 1996).

Despite initial alarm from the public health community regarding the relationship between the internet and STI outbreaks, research also demonstrates that people increasingly use the internet as an intermediary for health-related information. For instance, Gillett (2003) explores how people living with HIV/AIDS (PHAs) use the internet to seek out new information on medications and prevention, as well as to disseminate personal accounts of how new treatments have affected them. Kalichman et al. (2006) argue that AIDS service organizations (ASOs) that provide public internet services enable marginalized and underprivileged communities a means to access vital online health information. The internet also has appeal for those seeking information concerning sensitive or potentially embarrassing health matters. Notably, survey research by Berger et al. (2005) indicates that people suffering from stigmatized illnesses, including STIs, are especially likely to use the internet for health-related inquiries. This finding is supported by Bolding et al. (2004), who report that 84 per cent of HIV-positive men surveyed were likely to explore e-health information provided by M4M websites and chat rooms. There is also recognition that M4M websites offer an opportunity to discreetly reach men seeking men and distribute safer sex information. For example, both Klausner et al. (2004) and Tikkanen and Ross (2003) note that the internet is a useful tool for health educators to post cautionary advertisements and links to appropriate sexual health information. An online survey conducted by Salyers Bull et al. (2001) revealed that 61 per cent of men seeking men strongly supported using the internet to access STI/HIV prevention information; respondents also reported favouring different methods of access, including e-mail and interactive chat/message windows. Furthermore, Salyers Bull et al. argue that M4M websites are an ideal medium to promote risk reduction, as these venues attract specific subcultures that are often inaccessible to traditional prevention efforts.

Currently, many health researchers and educators are developing constructive strategies that make advantageous use of M4M websites as ICTs for effectively, yet unobtrusively, delivering health information. Examples include promising experimental programmes that have implemented online notification schemes, weblog bulletin boards, chat room health advisors, interactive 'gay' characters and sexualized games, and links to external health information resources (Flicker et al., 2006; Mimiaga et al., 2006; Rhodes et al., 2006). In some cases, those who operate M4M websites are actively collaborating with public health researchers to develop and refine intermediation strategies that more effectively address the specific needs of the diverse communities served by particular websites. One popular yet relatively new website, Manhunt.net, has even received accolades for its active role in working with private and public health professionals to promote sexual health and safety (Novak, 2004). However, as one might expect with many early-stage internet technologies intended to modify health outcomes, as yet there has been little opportunity to conduct follow-up research exploring actual use and efficacy.[3] Within this context, the role of M4M websites as intermediaries between health information and human interaction remains underdeveloped.

Exploring the use of M4M health initiatives by gay men

This project draws on the experiences of 21 individual interviews with gay men living in Toronto, Ontario who regularly use one or more of the following popular M4M websites: www.gay.com, www.mygaydar.com, www.men4sexnow.com, and www.manhunt.net. During the interviews the men were asked to describe their use of health information online: how often they used the internet to seek health information; whether they were familiar with the health services available on M4M websites; whether they trusted such information and found it useful; and the extent to which they seek out and incorporate the information into their sexual lives. While interviewees ranged in age from 20 to 52 years, most were between 20 and 36 years of age. Interviewees primarily discussed their use of four broadly described ICT intermediaries: online notification services, health advisories and information links, educational avatars and sexualized games, and interactive chat and online educators.

The four online intermediaries that are briefly profiled below have been produced specifically to disseminate health information intended to influence the sexual behaviour of men seeking men. They range from least to most interactive and personal; some are passive tools of larger intermediary structures, while others facilitate direct information exchange among parties. Online notifications are considered public service websites; they operate as part of official public health mandates or are affiliated with non-profit organizations. Health information links are technically located on private M4M websites, however the redirect takes online users to external web pages with official public health information, such as homepages for Health Canada or the Center for Disease Control in North America. Sometimes the information links are internal to M4M websites, in which case moderators provide abridged or paraphrased versions of public health information with links or citations to the official source. At present, educational avatars (animated people and things) and sexualized games (interactive modules) are largely pilot projects that have been initiated by public health agencies; they target youth and, in particular, gay and lesbian teens (one example is mysexycity.com). Chat room educators, by contrast, typically work for local health organizations in collaboration with private M4M websites. Some work specifically in chat rooms associated with the city of employment, while others rotate among regional chat rooms. Similar to public health workers who distribute condoms or safe sex information, chat room educators perform a comparable service online.

Online notification services

Non-profit and public health organizations have developed online notification websites as a discreet method by which people who have contracted an STI can anonymously inform recent sexual partners of the need to seek testing. One example, inSPOT.org, consists of a parent website with links to different major cities, from which visitors can send electronic cards to partners cautioning them of potential exposure to an STI. The warning is accompanied by information on symptoms and referrals to nearby clinics where the individual can seek testing. In this instance the ICT medium is asynchronous, impersonal and static, as opposed to synchronous and interactive. Since the inception of notification services, there has been doubt as to whether web users would send anonymous STI warnings to sexual partners. After all, even though the notification is anonymous, many men will have little difficulty identifying of the sender. However, according to Mimiaga et al. (2006), this method has been used successfully in Boston to notify sexual partners who, in turn, have sought medical testing and services. Notification is considered effective and credited with helping prevent wider STI transmission.

In contrast, the men I interviewed all expressed apprehension or scepticism about online notification services, citing concerns over privacy and embarrassment. They believe that partners can easily identify who sends an online notification.

> I'd be too embarrassed to [send an online notification] to someone I knew ... maybe for just a trick, but not, like, a regular fuck buddy. C'mon they'd totally know!

Those who were sceptical about online notifications tend to view the approach as impractical. Specific reasons include not keeping track of the online contact information of casual partners; alternatively, some men prefer to inform regular partners in person or not at all, assuming the individual will find out soon enough.

> [I] hate to say it, but I doubt people would go to the trouble [of sending a notification]. We'd like to think we would, but I seriously doubt it ... I mean, who even keeps track of all the guys you meet online and could find them again, plus lots of the handles [online usernames] are too much alike, anyway.

This statement expresses one of the practical difficulties with notification websites. Men who use the website to meet multiple anonymous partners are unlikely to keep track of contact information; men with regular partners opt to notify people in person. There was little variation among interviewees concerning notification sites. It should be noted, however, that none of the respondents had ever used this type of resource; likewise, none had previously received an online notification. I was unable to locate a link to an online notification service on any of the four popular M4M websites commonly referred to in this study, though such services are easily found using a basic online search. Perhaps the lack of immediate access via M4M websites also helps to explain their lack of use and popularity among this group of respondents. When further probed on this issue, however, respondents noted that their scepticism made them loath to seriously consider, much less explore, online notification sites.

Health advisories and information links

Homepage advisories and links to STI and other health information are relatively common to M4M websites, though they vary in emphasis and quality. Often they are a collaborative effort between public health organizations supplying information and website moderators that provide links as a free service to their members. Their intended benefit is to supply an informative resource that is both convenient and inviting for those who either read the advertisement by chance or actively seek it out. Some are a central focus for specific websites, are recurrent and are accompanied by attractive images; for other sites, information advisories are less common and require a concentrated effort to both find and navigate. The information is fixed instead of interactive, and therefore the links more accurately function as tools of intermediaries as opposed to interactive agents or structures of change. Like the notification services, these ICTs are asynchronous and can be impersonal. Those described as 'less' impersonal, however, are typically hosted by a M4M website as opposed to those that are only accessible by using a general search engine. Most interviewees report being aware that M4M websites often have online health information resources, and are confident the information is both current and accurate.

> I've looked at some of the links to safe sex information ... by clicking on the red ribbon and stuff. Most of it is stuff that I know, but haven't actually spent much time reading it all. I just know there's lots of different information, which is cool that it's there.

> Yeah, I know of those [advisory links]. Probably they do it for liability reasons – LOL. Glad it's there, though ... [I] Wouldn't hesitate to use it if I needed to.

Respondents almost unanimously acknowledged the presence of M4M online health advisories, but only a few have explored them. Some interviewees also noted that while they know about such services, they had since become part of the 'standard scenery' of the webpage or blended in, and are therefore typically ignored. Nevertheless, the respondents acknowledged awareness of the links and understanding of their long-term availability. The comments suggest that users often expect these advisories to offer only standard safer-sex information. Although these advisory links have been produced as generic and stable information sources, they sometimes lack practical allure which in turn inhibits regular or sustained use.

Respondents frequently mentioned the M4M website Manhunt (www.manhunt.net). Of the popular M4M websites discussed here, Manhunt is the most well known and widely used among interviewees. Manhunt is relatively new. Based in Massachusetts, it nevertheless sponsors many local events in Toronto, and regularly advertises in community newspapers, flyers, at nightclubs and bars, bathhouses, billboards and even on posters in the Wellesley subway station in the heart of the Toronto's gay community.

> I like Manhunt's format. A lot! I'm all about Manhunt, and not just because of the men on it. It's local so it's friendly and inviting. It has [links] to safe sex and testing resources. I know some of the people involved with creating the site, so I know the information is good information and I would definitely trust it.

Interviewees who regularly use Manhunt describe a pro-sex environment and a relatively diverse community of members, and recall seeing regular health advisories and information links. They describe this website as local, familiar, unobtrusive and easy to navigate. As the previous interviewee suggests, these positive qualities are combined with a level of comfort and trust towards the health information and advocates affiliated with this website. In this case, direct affiliation with the host site detracts from perceptions that the online advisories are impersonal, thus improving their function as informational tools. These findings are consistent with Rhodes' (2004) study of online STI interventions, which concludes that successful strategies result, in part, from an established relationship with regular users. Similarly, the importance of rapport is reminiscent of the recommendation by Salyers Bull et al. (2001) that effective ICT health strategies be able to cater to specific, local subpopulations.

Educational avatars and sexualized games

Combining educational avatars and interactive learning aids is another ICT approach to health promotion that has been produced by public health researchers for use on M4M websites. The avatars and information strategies discussed here have been designed specifically for M4M websites and are generally geared towards gay and bisexual youth. They use ethnically diverse characters and sexualized narratives; the goal is first to provide information, and later test knowledge and retention rates using interactive exercises. The interactive nature of the ICT mimics synchronous communication, while the illustrative content contributes to the perception that the technology is personal. On the downside, these technologies usually require advanced browsers and high-speed access, which limit distribution to the intended audience.[4] Interviewees in my study expressed mixed feelings about the potential of this technology; their reservations range from descriptions of such strategies as puerile to concerns about their practicality.

> I see those [avatars] all the time in community newspaper ads and, I think, on websites as well. I only know of them, I've never actually used one. I don't go on to play games; I go on to hook up.

> Yeah, I guess they're ... helpful if you're, like, a teen or something. I don't know personally, but it seems more like a novelty thing than actually useful. I could be wrong, I don't know. It just seems that way.

These quotes are typical among interviewees who generally perceived the avatar strategy as childish or felt the strategy might be initially entertaining but quickly suffer from waning novelty. Others expressed hesitation about exploring the external links for fear of inviting pop-up windows, receiving spam or, in extreme cases, causing their computer to 'crash' (especially where interactive websites are concerned). It should be noted, however, that the majority of the respondents are outside the adolescent age bracket for which this tool is designed and intended. Yet, even those who are critical of the websites acknowledged their potential for younger men seeking men.

Interestingly, the two youngest interviewees are less critical. They felt that the avatars and interactive ICTs possess definite potential for youth.

> First of all, those guys are hot, or images or whatever they are. They're hot. I'm laughing, but I'm serious. And they're campy and fun because I think you can make guys mount each other, so it seems like they'd be perfect for 'queens' that live online.

> I can see how they could be popular. I don't know too many younger guys that will spend a lot of time reading over really thick medical advice about safe sex or what to do or what to look out for ... and as long as it seems accurate to them it's probably as good as anything else.

These interviewees provided a different perspective on the perceived impracticalities suggested in the earlier set of statements. They note that the specific content of the avatars and interactive websites is both inviting and useful for the intended audience and contrasted the accessibility of the health and sexual information with the perceived complexity of other online health resources. Their comments are consistent with the results of a study of youth perspectives on the internet and online health initiatives, such as avatars and learning aids. Flicker et al. (2004) concluded that online health information that is developed and marketed specifically for youth is likely to be successful with this age group.

Interactive chat and online educators

Many M4M websites allow health professionals and community activists to create online profiles and advertise their availability as information sources. Trained health advocates are typically online at peak hours of popularity, advertising their presence and answering health-related questions posed by users. In my study, the synchronous, interactive nature of this strategy was favoured by the interviewees, contradicting previous research suggesting that synchronous online interventions are perceived as inaccurate and lacking privacy (Salyers Bull et al., 2001).[5] Interviewees felt that these resources are unobtrusive and possess legitimacy because they are integrated into the parent website, employ real people and provide person-to-person communication.

> So I got burned [gonorrhoea] by this guy. I knew what it was, right, by the feeling and the discharge – totally gross. I knew I had to get it looked at, right, but I was just hoping I could get [medication] without going to a doctor. Anyway, I just IM'd [instant messaged] one of those online social workers and asked what the easiest thing to do was. I ended up having to go to the doctor, which I knew I would, but they were still helpful ... and told me not to wait around and where the easiest place I could go was. It was all quick and easy.

Consistent with Wyatt et al.'s description of effective helpers (this volume, chapter 1), interviewees described these services as helpful and non-judgemental. The direct affiliation of health professionals with the M4M website is also viewed favourably. Likewise, some noted that the perceived professionalism helps assuage fears that information may not be held in confidence.

> Gay.com has lots of the online health people that you can ask questions. I don't know if they're doctors or nurses, but I know they're trained and provide accurate information. Plus, they're endorsed by the site ... not like those annoying pop-up windows.

> I've tried to chat with them before to see what they're all about. They're friendly, but they let you know they're there to answer real questions for people and not chit-chat around. They're sort of weird, but it's not like I think they're eavesdropping on me or judging me.

These statements convey a feeling that the online health educators possess authority and, consequently, that the information they communicate is legitimate. Interviewees also understood that these specialists are regularly available to answer questions or concerns, suggesting that the strategy has a lasting benefit for information consumers. Together, these findings suggest that the use of this combination of human and technical strategy for information provision on M4M websites accomplishes the important task of providing timely and effective, yet unobtrusive, information.

There are also instances in which men solicit options for 'safer unprotected' sex from chat room educators. This is a potentially volatile development given the often tense climate surrounding efforts to expand beyond traditional safe-sex literature and endorse unconventional harm-reduction techniques.

> There's more to sex than just using a condom or not. I know people that have asked them about barebacking [intentional unprotected anal intercourse] options. They probably don't encourage barebacking, but if you're gonna do it then you're gonna do it ... so I guess they may as well help out with [options that help reduce the risk].

Here, the respondent uses a second-hand example to allude to a dilemma that frequently occurs when personal sexual desire comes into conflict with public messages about safe sex. In such instances, people find themselves negotiating between two dichotomous situations: completely protected intercourse and completely unprotected intercourse. For many people, however, sex is not so compartmentalized. Speaking to this struggle over technical purpose versus online content, another interviewee recollects past efforts at providing harm reduction to the public.

Some years ago, [a local AIDS service organization] sponsored community speaking events aimed specifically at encouraging public discussion of barebacking. The idea was that people are doing it, so let's engage the issue responsibly rather than simply saying 'don't do it' and then thinking safe sex had been accomplished ... I would like to see [chat room educators] be able to fulfil a similar function.

The respondent offers this comparison as a reminder that sex without the use of a condom has been candidly and responsibly discussed without being seen to carelessly endorse high-risk behaviour. The noted success leads him to believe online health strategies have similar potential. Given the expanse of their technological reach and increasing hours of operation, the possibility for chat room educators to contribute to harm reduction strategies is worth consideration. Similarly, Rhodes (2004) finds that chat room health educators fulfil a broad range of needs, including specific questions around 'safer' barebacking practices. M4M online educators, therefore, offer a forum that permits people to ask about sexual practices that are considered extra-normative – practices they may be less likely to ask health professionals face-to-face. That said, this is an instance where the intended use of an online health strategy comes into conflict with a creative application of the technology.

Online health intermediaries within the circuit of culture

du Gay et al. (1997) and Hall (1997) outline a circuit of culture, which, they argue, can and should be used to analyse cultural products, or artefacts, and the origins of their creation. The framework is based on the articulation of distinct yet interacting processes that form linkages, which can prove temporary or enduring. These connections ultimately shape the unique cultural identity of an artefact, as well as significantly inform our individual role or collective understanding of the creation and use of cultural products.

Among the processes in the 'circuit' are instances of production, consumption and formation of identity. While cultural artefacts are typically embedded at inception with some intended meaning, ultimately meaning is the result of complicated processes and interactive, often unpredictable, relationships (du Gay et al., 1997). I apply this framework to understand how M4M websites have developed as a cultural artefact of technology. Their production and consumption occur in the context of complex, interacting relationships within the larger circuit of culture. The circuit in question is an example of a link between the commodification of sex and public health reasoning. After all, M4M websites were not originally created as vehicles for public health information, but as businesses produced to generate revenue for the website owners. The use of these websites by public health organizations as education intermediaries is an outcome of the articulation of production, consumption and regulation processes specific to this cultural artefact. As artefacts, they are unstable and changing hybrid spaces that mix desire and commodification of sex with health information. Men who frequent these sites are consumers who actively seek sex, but may also pair this use with an engagement of online health information. Thus, applying the framework of the circuit of culture to these findings lends insight into the use of M4M websites to disseminate and access sexual health information.

The online health intermediary strategies discussed rely on basic knowledge and access to innovative online technology. In each case, both the graphics and functions are produced by public health organizations often working in tandem with M4M website moderators. The health technologies are therefore produced in collaboration by public and private entities with a specific strategy in mind: they are encoded with meanings intended to cater to a target audience, namely men seeking men online.

Despite being key processes of the cultural circuit, however, production strategy and encoding are dependent on other aspects of the process, which make product consumption unstable. The data show that the use and consumption of online health information are neither passive experiences nor forgone conclusions for men seeking men. For example, respondents often cited Manhunt as a favourite M4M website. Their reasons for this preference varied from the website's local roots to a personal knowledge or familiarity with the moderators. In the latter case, the connection to production translated into identification with the product and personal investment in the outcome. This process bears a striking resemblance to the workings of the circuit of culture described above. In contrast, respondents report being suspicious of online notification services which, in turn, made them reticent to explore this online service. Users frequently describe online notifications as impersonal, which also contributes to a feeling of distrust. In each case, the goals and outcome of the production cycle are superseded by hesitation on the part of users to trust the source of creation. Likewise, inability among users to identify with the cultural product inhibits consumption from the outset. In contrast, the synchronous and interactive ICTs are frequently described as a friendly and trustworthy means of accessing STI information. The men in question actively interpret the websites within a context of their daily use and personal histories; they are not automata who follow blindly the goals of production, making it difficult to predict individual patterns of consumption.

The capacity of online notifications and information links as intermediaries is limited because they function more as tools than as operators causing change. By this I mean that the asynchronous structure of these online strategies limits the interactivity of a relationship between producer and consumer as well as the potential for creative use. As a result, the men I interviewed described them as less desirable and used the services less. In contrast, the interactive online strategies – and in particular, chat room educators – more frequently function as active, innovative agents because they mediate real-time dialogue between health community representatives and men seeking men online. That these ICTs are frequently described by users as trustworthy and readily accessible increases the potential of accomplishing their intended production goal. For instance, a frequent criticism of online search engines is that the sheer volume of information is often overwhelming and difficult to evaluate, even for people with some knowledge of a given topic. However, in a study of adolescent online health information use, Gray et al. (2005) note that online communities often help establish the credibility of professional health sources. The significance of their finding is especially compelling in a youth context, where the breadth of online information is frequently an obstacle and the topic of inquiry is potentially sensitive. The data presented in this research indicate that the health intermediary role served by online educators partially resolves this issue helping to establish the expertise of the source and trustworthiness of the information product.

Existing or future online health initiatives are likely to achieve similar success to the extent that they decrease the perceived social distance between producer and intended audience. Clearly, credibility and rapport are not guaranteed through production alone. Rather, they are invoked through the cycle of production and consumption, which in turn relies primarily on the mode of delivery. Moreover, as Rhodes (2004) notes, establishing trust initially requires considerable time investment on the part of online educators. In the examples above, intermediary strategies that were personalized and accomplished a measure of rapport were also the most preferred sources of health-related information by the target group.

The kind of health information provided for user consumption on M4M websites is cause for potential debate. Among health researchers and mainstream media alike, a lasting concern has been men who explicitly use these websites to seek out and arrange unprotected sexual encounters. Many M4M websites have resources specifically established to accommodate individual users interested in finding partners for unprotected sex, such as bareback-themed chat rooms. There is debate over whether these websites condone unprotected sex and so encourage an active culture of barebacking among men seeking men (Carballo-Dieguez and Bauermeister, 2004). In light of this ongoing debate, some argue that public health information and online interventions should strictly adhere to the safest, medically proven prevention strategies. However, Mykhalovskiy et al. (2004) caution that public health has a history of regulating people's sexuality. They argue against the traditional 'compliance model' of health service delivery, which privileges medical knowledge and control over patients' personal experiences in daily decision-making. Some interviewees openly discuss the reality of negotiating protected and unprotected intercourse. For them, much of the readily available safe-sex information conflicts with the reality of their regular sexual encounters. Instead, interactive online health resources provide credible yet nuanced information about safer sex that is otherwise difficult to locate. Under these circumstances the data indicate that consumption of online health information is not passive or 'compliant', but occurs through creative engagement that uses a health technology to negotiate medical knowledge in the service of lived experience and real-world decision-making concerning sexual practice.

On a related note, research by Davis et al. (2006) suggests that many HIV-positive men use the internet to engage in serosorting (finding HIV-positive sexual partners for unprotected sex). Doing so, they argue, helps HIV-positive men avoid both the subtle and overt stigma that is often directed at sexually active HIV-positive men. Furthermore, 84 per cent of HIV-positive men who frequent M4M websites report a willingness to use chat room health educators (Bolding et al., 2004). Extrapolating beyond these findings, one might reason that the kind of health information sought by some HIV-positive men falls beyond the purview of standard safe-sex prevention messages but is still vital to their health and well-being.[6] While some will undoubtedly frown at this prospect by arguing that it encourages risky behaviour, the reality of this interest among M4M users suggests that online educators operating in this capacity are offering a beneficial health service. Rather than relying on the same old safe-sex messages and operating from the assumption that people will passively consume information and then practise protected sex, it behooves online educators to engage with people about more complex areas of sexual practice that occur at the interface of desire and self-regulation. The realization that ICTs afford a public site where health information and services can be widely disseminated and privately accessed is an opportunity that should be more fully explored. Doing so not only invokes the iterative potential of the circuit of culture thus refining the eventual product, but also better develops the function of M4M websites as health intermediaries. For instance, Wyatt et al. (2005) explore the notion of 'warm experts', a concept used to identify individuals with technical expertise who provide instruction or guidance to the technical novice. They employ the term in an internet context to explore how people use online resources as intermediaries to locate and make sense of complicated health information.

The intermediary function of interactive online health advisors can also be compared to warm experts. These online operators are trusted resources that many men are able to comfortably contact for information ranging from mundane to delicate sexual matters. These warm experts are available to answer general questions about STIs or refer users to specific external web links. Alternatively, they can serve as a resource for interpreting complex information and helping users to work through context-specific situations, as with the example above. The practical benefit of these experts is diminished when they are limited to providing only the 'safest', officially sanctioned health information produced for public consumption. While they may operate in a fashion that is ideal from the perspective of the producers of public health information, their regulation hinders ideal use for some consumers. The benefit of these resources to the consumer inevitably expands when these experts are allowed flexibility to engage with a diverse range of online health queries, even those inquiring about sex that is to some extent classified as 'risky.' Thus, the actual experiences of these men indicate that M4M websites are not simply used as conduits for accessing fixed knowledge in commodity form, which is then dutifully applied as intended in safe sex applications. Rather, as health intermediaries these online strategies operate as negotiated terrains where information is interpreted and incorporated into people's lives in sometimes unanticipated ways.

Finally, processes of production and consumption are beset by regulation. According to du Gay et al. (1997) and Hall (1997), cultural artefacts inadvertently affect cultural life by blurring the distinctions between the public and private. In turn, institutions frequently attempt to regulate access to or control the use of artefacts; as a result, concerns around ethics often arise. M4M websites have been under the threat of regulation since health science research linked them with outbreaks of syphilis

(McFarlane et al., 2000; Chiasson et al., 2003). Similarly, they have been identified as sites of control by which health information can be disseminated (Klausner et al., 2000; Tikkanen and Ross, 2003). In each case, ethical questions concerning privacy have come to the forefront of discussion (Salyers Bull et al., 2001). Use of M4M websites as mechanisms for health intervention necessitates respecting the confidentiality of website members and protecting the identity of users seeking health information and services. It is equally important that the interventions operating on existing M4M websites do not deter current or future users from accessing these venues. The fact that some interviewees express concern about privacy and regulation indicates that the ethics of online health interventions continue to be an important topic of discussion. However, it is also important to note the interviewees express more concern about the prospect of being directly contacted without consent by unknown or obscure entities than about being identified or sought by educators affiliated with familiar websites. Thus, while use of M4M personals sites as health intermediaries should proceed with caution, it should also be done with the knowledge that responsible production on the part of educators can encourage responsible consumption of important sexual health information among the target audience.

Acknowledgement

This research was supported by Action for Health. Interview and transcription facilities were provided by the Qualitative Research and Resource Center, York University. I also want to thank Lorna Erwin and Eric Mykhalovskiy for their editorial suggestions.

Notes

1. For example, Eysenbach and Jadad (2001) envisage the confluence of digital and information technologies as ushering in an era of consumer health informatics, wherein the online public has unprecedented access to information that enables active, informed involvement in health decision-making processes. While Eysenbach and Jadad acknowledge the many obstacles that continue to impede the shared decision-making ideal, they also outline potential directions for future academic research in this area.
2. Localized websites and chat rooms cater to a specific geographic locale (e.g. a 'TorontoM4M' chat room).
3. One notable exception is Rhodes' (2004) study of a chat room intervention introduced by an AIDS service organization (ASO) to provide health information to men seeking men online.

4. According to Skinner et al. (2003), 'functionality' is one of the key factors influencing the quality of youth internet access. E-health potential, they argue, is especially limited for youth living in small urban or rural communities with low bandwidth or few internet access sites. Geographically isolated youth who must rely on dial-up internet access are therefore less likely to benefit from certain ICTs, such as educational avatars and sexualized games.

5. The data reflect a sample of online users in general and not specifically men seeking men, which may help account for the disparity.

6. While unprotected sex among seroconcordant HIV-positive partners does not run the risk of new transmission, there is still risk of co-infection of other STIs or a more virulent strain of HIV. Therefore, online health initiatives still remain a vital source of important information specific to the HIV-positive community, especially when one considers that the sexual lives and health of PHAs remain largely unaddressed outside of physician–patient relationships. Moreover, the active sexual lives of PHAs is a subject that remains fraught with public disapproval and entrenched in personal stigma for many. With all this in mind, it is easy to recognize how interactive health services hosted by M4M websites and chat rooms are especially appealing for many PHAs.

8

Between the Clinic and the Community: Pathways for an Emerging e-Health Policy in the Remote First Nations of Northwestern Ontario

Adam Fiser and Robert Luke

The Sioux Lookout Zone of Northwestern Ontario, Canada is home to 24 First Nations communities of Cree-, Oji-Cree- and Ojibway-speaking peoples. Their land is about as far from the urban landscape as one can get in Ontario, a swathe of boreal forest extending from the edge of the 50th parallel to the sub-arctic shores of Hudson Bay. The total population of less than 25,000 amounts to about 0.1 persons per square kilometre over a territorial expanse the size of France. Mobility to and from these communities is difficult and expensive, with light aircraft and watercraft the primary modes of transportation except between January and March, when the waterways freeze and become temporary highways for long-haul transport, snowmobiles and 4 × 4 vehicles.

In the mid- to late 1800s many of these communities continually migrated around family trap lines and bush camps, remnants of the former staple economy studied by Innis (1930). The ancestors of today's Sioux Lookout Zone First Nations traded furs and other goods with the Hudson's Bay and Northwest trading companies. In the early 1900s they began to take treaty with the Crown and settle on reserve land, many out of fear that an encroaching railway system would ruin their economy and habitat (Morrison, 1986). Physicians also began to periodically visit the reserve settlements to offer treaty-based services and take accounts of the population.

Today, regional unemployment is approximately 37 per cent, and federal government services dominate the job market on the 'reserves' occupied by the First Nations communities. The mid- to larger-sized communities have Northern Stores which sell a wide variety of consumer goods, from groceries to all-terrain vehicles. For residents of the larger communities, electricity, water treatment/sewerage and telephone services are late twentieth- and early twenty-first-century additions. Like the winter roads and the supply chain of goods, keeping these services in operation requires local initiative, creative enterprise and goodwill.

The decline of the traditional staple economy and the parallel encroachment of the state in Aboriginal affairs have left lasting impressions on these communities. Over 130 years[1] of colonial influence in the affairs of First Nations peoples have reshaped their environments and restructured their societies. For example, family trap lines have been eroded by the encroachment of state-subsidized forestry, mining and energy concerns;[2] and residential schooling[3] separated children from their families and demanded that they assimilate non-indigenous languages and cultures. Hereditary and clan-based forms of governance were supplanted by non-indigenous forms of bureaucracy that have evolved into today's governance system.

Attempts continue to redress the historical events that have influenced First Nations communities and to foster Aboriginal self-governance. Most First Nations governing groups, or Bands, now manage their affairs through an elected Chief and Council with support from local Band Office staff in a variety of portfolios, including public administration, education, health and public utilities. Bands pass resolutions and direct fiscal spending; however, they report to the various Government of Canada departments and ministries from which they receive funding. This governance system depends on both the capacity of the local communities and the state to honour its fiduciary[4] commitments to the First Nations. Mirroring the Band Offices' various functions, nearly all the major federal departments and a number of ministries at the provincial level – education and health in particular – maintain an Aboriginal portfolio. Of significance in this dual system is the work of mediators in the First Nations and government agencies who are able to coordinate community policy with the policies of the state.

Beyond the high cost of living in the Sioux Lookout Zone, the challenges in First Nations communities are many. More than half the people who live there are under the age of 20, and their elders, the traditional keepers of knowledge and community policy, have diminished to a small fraction of the population. Between these demographic cohorts are the adults of age to govern and lead but who face daunting circumstances, including the emotional scars of residential schooling and forced relocation, socio-economic depression, drastic changes to traditional ways of life, heteronomous bureaucracies located hundreds of kilometres away and an increasing demand for their communities' natural resources. Local mediators who can productively manage such areas of potential conflict are in great demand to work in the Band Offices and NGOs particular to the First Nations' social economy, such as tribal councils, child and family services, education facilities and health organizations that support the implementation of community policy within the bounds of the state.

Among the most salient points in the contemporary configuration of this community structure is the status of remote First Nations health care and its delivery. Information and communications technologies (ICTs) have become increasingly integrated within Ontario's health care system and provincial and federal bureaucrats have become enthusiastic believers in the possibility of enhanced efficiencies through e-health. As the broader health care system adapts to e-health and ICT-intensive initiatives such as electronic health records, patient-managed care and telemedicine, the ways in which communities operate in Northwestern Ontario will change. Since 1998, the First Nations of the Sioux Lookout Zone have worked hard, not only by preparing for the impact of new technologies, but by taking steps to shape the local systems through which e-health will operate. Their efforts to translate federal and provincial e-health policies into community policies provide the focal points for this chapter.

A case of dual health care systems

The First Nations of northern Ontario enact a community-based approach to care and a holistic theory of health that focuses on the well-being of the individual as a member of a community connected to the land and its history (Berkes, 1999). This method of health care, whether initiated by families, social circles or special status groups, includes remedies for the emotional, spiritual and mental layers of being that envelop the physical (Struthers, 2000; Wilson, 2001). Community survival has depended on this deep ecological view of the individual's well-being (Adelson, 2000), a view similar to that described of Aboriginal peoples in Australia (see Simpson et al., this volume).

Modern (Western) medicine has a more recent history among the First Nations. Under a federal policy that began in 1930, Health Canada established health clinics in First Nations communities to support visiting clinicians (primarily nurses, who began to offer services in 1922). Most health clinics, or nursing stations as they were originally called, now have at least one full-time nurse who manages primary care and coordinates the schedules of visiting physicians and specialists (Seaby, 2002). In 1962, Health Canada began to support the integration of clinical and community-based health care, funding para-professionals in the communities to work as health representatives. Similar to the Aboriginal Health Workers described by Simpson et al. (this volume), these community health representatives provide an important mediating role between the clinic and the communities' own healing traditions, working in the language and cultural idiom of their communities and offering a set of (largely uncodified) basic clinical skills (McCulla, 2004; Hammond, 2006). As with other para-professional roles in the First Nations, the skills acquired by community health representatives are learned largely by doing and through peer support (Caplette, 1999; McCulla, 2004: 41).

In the 1980s, Health Canada began to transfer programme funds directly to First Nations Bands (Health Canada, 2005; First Nations and Inuit Health Branch, 2006). This saw the emergence of First Nations health authorities instituted by Bands to direct programme funds towards community health policy. In a parallel move to support community policy, Health Canada expanded the para-professional roles it funds, creating programmes for community health workers (CHWs). CHWs are hired by First Nations authorities to work in the clinic and community at large to help their fellow citizens with a range of health-related issues such as child care, elder care, fitness, nutrition, addictions, mental health, crisis work and more. Many of these community health workers focus on healing the scars of forced cultural assimilation and remedying the effects of significant changes in lifestyle on diet and occupation. They are as much in tune with the historical dynamics of community well-being as they are with the emotional, mental and spiritual dimensions of patient health.

Although both depend on Health Canada programme funds, the roles of clinicians and community health workers represent culturally distinct views on health care. Of these dual systems, the former is grounded in a medical tradition and clinical profession that privileges biophysical diagnosis and treatment. Unlike the communities' systems of survival, this is high-cost, high-tech health care that demands a full complement of equipment and supporting pharmaceutical, physiotherapeutic, transport and patient information systems. In contrast, the community systems are largely social and focused on behavioural change rather than invasive treatment. They demand far fewer material resources and create much less impact on the individual's physical constitution and his or her environment. In distinguishing between these health care systems we do not intend to propose that one is better than the other or that one system satisfies all the needs of the First Nations. As they exist today, the systems are dual yet complementary components of health care (cf. Pong et al., 1995; Kirmayer et al., 2003). Provided that access can be implemented in a manner that is consistent with community policy, First Nations patients want access to both.

In portraying a dual health care system in the First Nations we are wary of creating the impression of stasis. There are macro-changes at play that appear to be restructuring the rules of both types of health care. Today, the clinical and community-based components of the Aboriginal health care system are becoming integrated into one emerging e-health network. The hegemonic rationale[5] within the bureaucracies of Health Canada and the Ontario's Ministry of Health is to utilize ICTs to mitigate the costs of distributed health care between the remote and metropolitan areas, and to enhance First Nations' access to health care, without negatively affecting the quality of that care.

Based on what we have seen and heard, community health workers and clinicians operating in the communities are excited about the prospects of greater access and improved care; but they also harbour concerns about ICTs. The emerging e-health systems should not compromise patient safety or create overwhelming demands on the capacities of clinicians and community health workers who have to manage the changing systems at the levels of personal health and community well-being.

e-Health in the Sioux Lookout Zone

In the late 1970s, the Sioux Lookout Zone hospital began experimenting with teleconferencing as well as slow-scan video for the transmission of X-ray images over telephone lines. The experiment was intended to connect nursing stations (in three First Nations) and Sioux Lookout with clinical staff in Toronto, but some enterprising community members and nurses also used the phones to connect patients convalescing away from home to their family (Dunn et al., 1980). In the mid-1990s, Health Canada implemented Merlin, an experimental satellite-based system that connected three remote nursing stations by ISDN video to the Sioux Lookout Zone hospital. It, too, was primarily an experiment in clinical communications. As early models of e-health, neither of these Zone experiments included First Nations input in their explicit design, and budgetary constraints forced Merlin to end after its pilot phase.

In 1998, a coalition of First Nations working with federal and provincial agencies under the leadership of Keewaytinook Okimakanak Tribal Council (KO)[6] began a seven-year project to build a broadband Wide

Area Network (WAN) to connect the 24 communities of the Sioux Lookout Zone (Ramirez et al., 2003; Fiser et al., 2006; Fiser and Clement, 2007). The WAN – K-Net – provides a range of voice, video and data-switching services over a hybrid terrestrial/satellite network. It regularly supports multipoint video and multimedia streaming in real time. Its management organization, KO's K-Net Services, also hosts a range of internet service provider (ISP) services for First Nations, including email, content management systems, instant messaging (IM) conferencing and more.

In 1998, KO responded to First Nations interest in telehealth by piloting a videoconference and remote heart monitoring application over K-Net, in partnership with the Communications Research Centre (Industry Canada), Health Canada, the Ottawa Heart Institute, Computing Devices Canada, and the Margaret Cochenour Memorial Hospital in the town of Red Lake (Northwestern Ontario). The application was positively evaluated and became part of the hospital's cardiological protocol. In 1999, KO initiated a telepsychiatry pilot with Health Canada, Nodin Counselling, the London Psychiatric Hospital and Virtual Professionals Incorporated. Counsellors, health professionals, and clients in Sioux Lookout and Red Lake used K-Net supported videoconferencing for therapeutic and professional development purposes. As models of e-health these first KO telehealth experiments demonstrated the possibility of a First Nations directed telehealth network.

Building from their previous experiments, in 2002, K-Net members launched KO Telehealth, also under the Tribal Council's leadership, which expanded to all 24 Zone communities by 2005 (Rowlandson, 2005). It is currently Canada's largest Aboriginal telemedicine pilot project and the first to be operated by a First Nations-owned network. Behind the scenes, this project exemplifies the kind of infrastructure development to which Health Canada, the province and corresponding levels of Aboriginal governance turn when deliberating the implementation of Aboriginal e-health policy.

KO Telehealth has undergone continual organizational change and, in mid-2007, was rebranded as KO Telemedicine.[7] At the time of writing, we had every reason to believe the project would continue but that certain elements of its programme, particularly the community-based health care components, were at risk of being underestimated and possibly misunderstood by policy-makers. In light of the dual health care systems model described above, our analysis concentrates on these community components and their particular needs within the emerging e-health macro-system.

KO Telehealth/Telemedicine

Currently, the First Nations Inuit Health Branch (FNIHB) of Health Canada dedicates resources to cover the operational costs of telemedicine and other e-health-related network sessions in the 24 Zone communities (plus one southern community). Telemedicine in the Zone also depends on a partnership between FNIHB, KO Telehealth/Telemedicine and the Ontario Telemedicine Network (OTN). The OTN connects K-Net to Ontario's e-health backbone, enabling health clinics in the 24 Zone First Nations to communicate with and access physicians and specialists from five hospitals in Ontario and Manitoba (including a variety of clinical specialists from potentially 70 different specialties over the

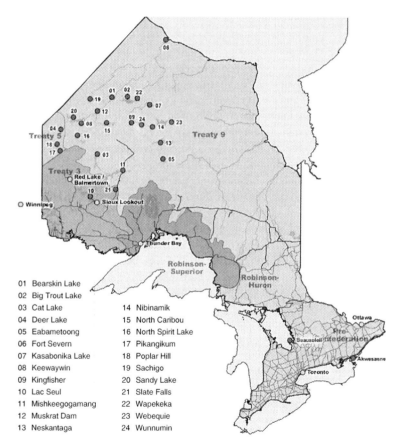

01	Bearskin Lake		
02	Big Trout Lake		
03	Cat Lake	14	Nibinamik
04	Deer Lake	15	North Caribou
05	Eabametoong	16	North Spirit Lake
06	Fort Severn	17	Pikangikum
07	Kasabonika Lake	18	Poplar Hill
08	Keewaywin	19	Sachigo
09	Kingfisher	20	Sandy Lake
10	Lac Seul	21	Slate Falls
11	Mishkeegogamang	22	Wapekeka
12	Muskrat Dam	23	Webequie
13	Neskantaga	24	Wunnumin

Figure 8.1 KO Telehealth/Telemedicine Network, communities, and Treaty areas

OTN). In terms of other network sessions shaping e-health policy, KO Telehealth/Telemedicine (KOTH/M) provides a variety of educational and information services in support of clinicians and community health workers based in the Sioux Lookout Zone.

From FNIHB Health Canada's policy perspective, KOTH/M's mandate was to mediate consultations between patients and clinicians (i.e. doctors and specialists) in distant locations. This narrow view of e-health is commonly known as telemedicine, which is basically the use of ICTs to enable medical interventions at a distance. Telemedicine does not, for example, include the use of ICTs for public health education or staff peer support in its definition, nor does it include the management of patient information systems or the use of search engines to retrieve health information. These other ICT-based systems fall under the more general heading of e-health, which also includes systems of organizational change related to enabling the effective use of ICT infrastructure.

To support telemedicine, KOTH/M's technical infrastructure was installed in each community's nursing station where patients would normally meet a staff nurse or visiting clinician. The technology associated with KOTH/M involves a retrofitted videoconferencing unit and television display, both fixed to a mobile cart. The unit can interface with a variety of peripheral diagnostic devices such as a remote heart monitor, a patient view cam (e.g. to capture digital images of dermal abrasions), an otoscope, tools for teleophthalmology and more. Each unit connects to the K-Net WAN via ethernet switch, receiving a dedicated portion of network bandwidth through an IP VLAN and network routing configuration managed by KO Tribal Council's K-Net Services[8] in cooperation with staff at the Ontario Telemedicine Network (OTN). Employees of the Tribal Council, under KOTH/M, schedule the consultations across the $24 + 1$ communities to optimize use of limited community bandwidth.[9]

Through telemedicine a physician or specialist consults with the patient from one of the urban hospitals or clinics networked with the OTN. The patient interacts with the clinician from his or her community's local health clinic, assisted by a nurse and community telehealth coordinator (CTC). The CTC is a para-professional hired by KOTH/M from the community who prepares the equipment (and may assist the remote physician). The attending staff nurse may observe or assist in the consult and manipulate the diagnostic tools on behalf of the physician. As part of Health Canada and OTN's broader telemedicine toolkit, the health clinics also utilize digital x-ray technology, which enables the transfer of images over the network and has substantially reduced waiting times for diagnosis (CraNHR, 2006a).

This description is only a partial model of KOTH/M's policy objectives. Other local systems promoted by KO Tribal Council and First Nations community policy include, on the community-based health care side, education and public health information sessions. Here the videoconferencing units are used by community health workers and other para-professionals to facilitate peer support and hold virtual seminars with distant clinics on various health issues. Moreover, KOTH/M has opened its broader interest seminars to the general public to help community members learn more about such issues as diabetes, child care and nutrition. It has also deployed videoconferencing to support social gatherings across the communities, for example, sponsoring semi-monthly luncheons for frail and elderly community members.

In its community policy context the KOTH/M pilot project is clearly more than an experiment in telemedicine. To be fair to Health Canada and the OTN, we acknowledge their use of education sessions to promote human resources development in the clinical and community-based systems. Moreover, we acknowledge that at the time of this study, FNIHB Health Canada supported KOTH/M through a transfer fund that (in addition to administrative costs) paid KO's K-Net Services a flat monthly rate per community to cover bandwidth charges and other network costs related to KOTH/M's use of the K-Net WAN[10] without distinguishing clinical sessions from other KOTH/M network activities, such as education or peer support. Our criticism is that telemedicine narrowly frames the bureaucratic policy perspective on what constitutes an effective use of KOTH/M, which leads to an underdevelopment of the system's complementary community-based e-health components and other potential applications.

How telemedicine frames KOTH/M

Telemedicine consultations are used primarily to replace face-to-face clinical consultations and follow-up visits, but are not intended as a substitution for emergency medical evacuations. Within these bounds KOTH/M forecast that between 15 and 20 per cent of consultations and follow-ups in the Sioux Lookout Zone could be accomplished through telemedicine (KO Telehealth Migration Workshop, 2002). From FNIHB Health Canada's perspective KOTH/M's future sustainability (beyond its pilot phase) depends on how it balances telemedicine's capital and operational costs with savings incurred by reductions in health-related travel. In the final evaluation of KOTH/M's pilot phase in 2006, the evaluators projected ongoing total costs for the programme at CAD $2.8 m/year

(CRaNHR, 2006a). They then estimated that with an annual utilization rate of 4,866 network sessions, savings from averted travel would be around CAD $4.2 m/year to create an estimated net savings of CAD $1.4 m/year. (The breakeven point was projected to be at 3,220 network sessions/year.) In comparison, the magnitude of costs incurred by health-related travel (without telemedicine) has been approximately four times higher than the projected ongoing cost of telemedicine. To put this in context, in fiscal year 2001/2, FNIHB Health Canada spent CAD $12.2 m on non-emergency, patient-related transport in the Sioux Lookout Zone.

Since 2003 the average number of monthly KOTH/M sessions has tripled and between April 2005 and March 2006 there were 2,752 network sessions. With respect to the projections of the 2006 breakeven analysis this total needs to be disaggregated for, of the 2,752 sessions, 1,187 were telemedicine consults (including telepsychiatry and teleopthalmology). The rest consisted of meetings, education sessions, family visits, demonstrations, training, tests and other uses of the video-conferencing equipment. Many of these other network sessions are clearly difficult to evaluate in terms of averted travel. They can, however, be assessed in terms of how they contribute to human resources development, administration and community well-being, but through a narrow telemedicine-based view of e-health their diverse values remain hidden. Keeping these values hidden poses problems for KOTH/M's sustainability for it will likely be more difficult to maintain KOTH/M's operations within a funding model narrowly framed by averted travel.

In negotiating KOTH/M's future sustainability, FNIHB and KO managers have discussed the allocation of operational funds from a FNIHB funding category called non-insured health benefits. Among other uses, these benefits fund non-emergency travel, enabling remote patients to use medical services that are not available on reserve. If it were to draw KOTH/M's funding base from non-insured health benefits, FNIHB would be clearly framing the system in terms of how it enhances patient access to clinical services that were previously unavailable on reserve, thus diminishing the need for non-emergency patient travel. Within this frame, education and other uses would be ancillary operations, permitted so long as a requisite number of telemedicine sessions were achieved (e.g. beyond KOTH/M's projected breakeven point).

Unfortunately, even if it enabled other network sessions to thrive, this sustainability model risks alienating First Nations patients. The non-insured health benefits that fund non-emergency medical-related travel are an important facet of the First Nations' health care experience and frame patients' perceptions of the quality of care they receive.

Community members associate this funding category with an effective health care system that includes physical access to a range of medical services in the nearest metropolitan areas. Aboriginal and federal policy analysts watching KOTH/M's emergence in the Zone have told us they fear community members may consider telemedicine to be a threat to quality of care if health care benefits are reduced.[11] Indeed, we have been told that since KOTH/M emerged in 2002, non-insured health benefits have drastically diminished due to cutbacks at FNIHB. Any sustainability model for KOTH/M, regardless of how narrowly it frames e-health, must therefore strike a careful balance between altering the health care benefits that communities have come to expect and delivering on the promises of an efficient and effective telemedicine system.

Within a more comprehensive vision of e-health, network sessions other than telemedicine must also have a value beyond averted patient travel. In an attempt to measure the potential worth of KOTH/M's non-clinical sessions, its pilot phase evaluators created an alternative model that included a distinct category called 'new telehealth' for which sessions such as education and training were estimated to create a value of approximately CAD \$3.2 m/year, based on projected savings in travel, accommodation and related administrative costs from a utilization rate of 4,866 sessions (CRaNHR, 2006a). As far as we know, FNIHB has chosen not to factor in a category comparable to 'new telehealth' in its assessment of KOTH/M. However, as we shall discuss in detail below, many FNIHB programmes are oriented towards community-based health care, supporting local Band Office staff and para-professionals. As community health workers and related para-professionals have adopted KOTH/M's videoconferencing facilities (and the K-Net WAN more generally) for training, peer support and other communications tasks, some important lessons have already been learned that should inform e-health policy and enrich the bureaucratic perspective's vision of KOTH/M's scope and value.

Community policy and local reactions

In 2002, researchers at KO Telehealth/Telemedicine conducted a series of focus groups with Zone First Nations to study their technology needs in the health care context (Report on the First Nations Telehealth Workshop, 2002: 6–8). They learned that community members envisaged a broad scope for KOTH/M, one that included telemedicine but went substantially beyond it. Respondents wanted KOTH/M's core and peripheral devices to be easy to use by the community-based para-professionals as well as by clinicians. They emphasized that KOTH/M should respond to each community's self-directed wellness priorities and include education and peer support programmes. They strongly felt that telemedicine will not succeed in the First Nations unless it can be shown that clinical consultations are private and secure for patients, and lead to added value beyond cost reductions in non-emergency medical travel. Finally, community members emphasized that e-health policy should be community-driven with appropriate regional, provincial and federal support to enhance citizen access to medical and health information services, including the enhancement of health-related employment opportunities for First Nations people.

Clinicians appear to share a number of the communities' concerns. Physicians and clinical specialists who responded to KOTH/M's final evaluation in 2006 agreed that telemedicine should be an add-on and never a complete substitute for face-to-face consultations (CRaNHR, 2006b). They were generally supportive of KO Telehealth, but questioned the demands telemedicine might place on nurses including demands on their time as well as for new ICT-related skills and training related to the operation of diagnostic equipment to assist specialists at a distance.[12] Nurses who responded to KOTH/M's 2006 evaluation were concerned that the nursing stations are not large enough to house the technical infrastructure. Some also wondered about patient reactions to telemedicine's video interface and its disruption of the 'normal' consultation's face-to-face interaction. Nevertheless, they welcomed the chance to enhance the clinical health care system with telemedicine and showed an interest in the new education and peer support opportunities that videoconferencing could offer.

Most of the clinicians in KOTH/M's 2006 evaluation agreed that the presence of a community health worker role was important to help establish community trust in telemedicine and manage the flow of work in emerging e-health systems. KO Telehealth was especially cognizant of the cultural need for a new mediator role in 2001 and created a job for community members to directly participate in the programme and support its clinical trials. This is the role of community telehealth coordinators.

A new (e-health) mediator enters the Zone

Under the KOTH/M model, before prospective community telehealth coordinators are accepted, they must undergo a certification process developed and instituted by KO Telehealth. Through this process CTCs learn a variety of tasks, including how to set up telemedicine equipment for clinical consults, how to guide consults, how to operate videoconferencing units for general meetings and how to promote KOTH/M to patients and the wider community. In this way the CTC role provides community members with opportunities to learn about and handle telemedicine and videoconferencing in order to help KOTH/M and its partners build e-health systems that community members will trust. At present, formal qualifications for the role are minimal. As with most community health worker roles, 'learning by doing' predominates and peer support is essential for effective job performance.

In terms of the community telehealth coordinators' own beliefs about the role, there is some evidence from research leading up to KOTH/M's 2006 evaluation that they are less interested in handling clinical systems than in enabling community-based health care (Ibanez, 2004). In an attempt to understand how they view different aspects of the job, KOTH/M's evaluators found that CTCs ranked highest overall time spent attending KOTH/M educations sessions and time spent with community health workers. Their lowest job rankings concerned 'working with physicians' (including manipulating peripherals during consultations) and 'promotion' (including encouraging community members to participate in telehealth) (Ibanez, 2004). There is lingering uncertainty over why these rankings occurred. It could be that some CTCs find the clinical setting technically challenging and socially unfamiliar. More fundamental value differences could also be shaping community beliefs in the purpose of the role.

Like community health workers and community health representatives, the community telehealth coordinators perceived themselves as mediators working between clinical and community-based understandings. They perceived their primary task as translating 'medical and technical concepts and clinical jargon to the clients, especially those of more advanced age, who are not fluent in English' (Ibanez, 2004: 5). Respondents told the KOTH/M evaluator that they considered this cultural aspect of their job to be the top community need related to their role within telehealth. CTCs also indicated a preference for team-building, not primarily with clinicians, but with other para-professionals (Ibanez, 2004: 5).

To be effective mediators the CTCs require opportunities to educate themselves regarding both the clinical and community-based health care systems. How they prefer to spend their work time appears to be skewed in favour of the community-based health care system. A possible reinforcement of this preference can be found in the frequency and duration of KOTH/M network sessions. In the final KOTH/M evaluation

(CRaNHR, 2006a), evaluators found that overall, clinical consultations comprised 42 per cent of 2,926 sessions, followed by education (19 per cent), training (18 per cent), administrative meetings (13 per cent) and demonstrations/systems tests/family visits (8 per cent). Although the frequency data suggest that clinical consultations were the dominant form of network session, in terms of the duration of network sessions (based on total minutes), education sessions amounted to 40 per cent, followed by clinical (26 per cent), meetings (21 per cent) and other sessions (5 per cent). While education sessions averaged about 107 minutes, clinical sessions averaged about 35 minutes.

As we understand their mediator role, CTCs normally participate in the set-up and take-down of clinical sessions. The intensity and extent of their participation may vary during actual diagnostic interventions at the patient end, and nurses are often present and may intervene. Education sessions, however, normally involve several CTCs for the full duration of a session, alongside a variety of community health workers and community health representatives (depending on session topics, personal preferences, and so on). In terms of time spent on the job, education sessions may have a greater influence on CTCs' interpretation of their roles than clinical sessions, especially considering the importance of 'learning by doing' in the CTC job role. These are clearly the network sessions in which CTCs and community health workers have the grreatest exposure to KOTH/M and the videoconferencing technology. The data suggest that KOTH/M's pilot project, more than merely increasing efficiencies in the clinical system, reflects and reinforces the notion of two systems of health care. CTCs straddle both systems and perceive themselves as mediators, but appear to find their most natural fit in the community-based health care system.

Is there a role conflict here? One problem is that the community-based health care system which takes up the majority of the CTC's time on the job and which appears to be prioritized by the CTCs in evaluations, has not received adequate attention by Health Canada. Education sessions became an official component of KOTH/M in 2004. An education coordinator position was created to support the community health workers' use of videoconferencing for education and peer support; but funds to maintain this role were not allocated from any of FNIHB Health Canada's community programmes. Instead, KOTH/M had to secure contract funds from the province's Ministry of Health. The contracts have been temporary and the available funds have not stretched far beyond supporting a single education coordinator for all 25 KOTH/M First Nations.

To help clarify the state of community telehealth coordinators' and community-health workers' needs, KOTH/M's education coordinator conducted a comprehensive community survey in 2006. The survey polled 51 community health workers and CTCs about their past and current experiences with education systems and revealed that only 27 per cent of the respondents had completed high school or any post-secondary education. Nevertheless, the majority of respondents indicated a desire to pursue continuing education, particularly diploma programmes related to health care and professional vocations, followed by certificate programmes related to community health and on-the-job training to further their careers. Given the limited resources that they can dedicate to education we are not certain that KOTH/M or its local collaborators can offer sufficient career support to help these individuals. With regard to their perceptions of training related directly to their roles as community health workers, community health representatives or CTCs, 33 per cent of the survey respondents indicated that they had not received adequate training (KO Telehealth, 2006). In terms of an emerging e-health curriculum, among the critical ICT-based learning needs listed by the respondents were basic computer training (office software) and networking. The majority of respondents also indicated a desire to participate in online instruction to pursue continuing education opportunities.

Although it funds and supports community-based health care, FNIHB Health Canada has not clearly defined its position on the role of ICTs in that paradigm, especially with regard to supporting the career development of community health workers. KOTH/M's activities in community education have had to emerge *ad hoc*, through provincial support, and it is unclear that the First Nations' education needs are being met since there have not been enough resources in place to develop local systems to help them track their progress and participation under the various KOTH/M-sponsored learning initiatives.

We believe that if FNIHB Health Canada wants to reinforce local appreciation for the clinical aspects of e-health to, among other objectives, improve the uptake of telemedicine, its change management strategy should be holistic and include resources and systems that address the community health workers' education and capacity needs. Community health care systems are strong cultural determinants of the First Nations' entire health care experience. Encompassing personal health and community wellness, they frame patients' perceptions of the quality of care. To be successfully integrated as a positive force in the First Nations' health care experience, e-health tools such as telemedicine need to be translated in terms of community health and be confidently endorsed by community health workers if they are to be taken up and owned by the communities.

As we write this chapter we have reason to believe that programme support along those lines could be forthcoming. In its 2007 compendium of Aboriginal services FNIHB lists capacity development as an important element of a successful Aboriginal e-health system, focusing specifically on:

> the sustainment of community health personnel at the regional and local level through education with the goal to improve health service delivery, health service planning and community health program development. It also addresses partnership with other government organizations and non-government organizations (NGO) to build e-health capacity in First Nations and Inuit communities.
>
> (2007: 67)

Education and the capacity needs of emerging e-health systems

Our position on e-health's emergence in the Sioux Lookout Zone is informed by research conducted in 2006 under the PePTalk-K-Net project, a collaboration between KO Tribal Council and Princess Margaret Hospital of Toronto funded by the Inukshuk fund.

Our research objective under the project was to work with Zone First Nations to learn how community health workers acquire and organize locally relevant health information. We wanted to understand their use of a range of ICTs, including videoconferencing and web-based information systems (such as search engines, content management systems, email, IM, and so forth).

K-Net Services archives nearly all of the education sessions conducted by KOTH/M. The result is an online media library replete with seminars and lectures conducted by local experts within a northern Ontario First Nations context. Preliminary encounters with a group of 17 CTCs and community health workers from the First Nations led us to explore the archived education and peer support sessions. We learned that the education sessions involve multiple KOTH/M communities and consist of CTCs and participating community health workers interacting by multipoint videoconference over a range of health topics such as diabetes, addictions, nutrition, crisis intervention, child care, elder care, tobacco control, mental health, occupational therapy, and so forth.

We were told that the sessions, often led by a local expert from the Sioux Lookout Zone, provide the participants with valued opportunities to expand their knowledge of a particular health issue relevant to their community work. We were also told that CTCs and community health workers value these encounters for the opportunity to become acquainted with peers in other communities who are working on similar health issues.

The general quality of the videoconferences we reviewed was diverse.[13] Some groups in the sessions were thoroughly immersed in the new medium, interweaving edited video clips and/or presentation slides in their real-time presentations. Others had difficulty operating the videoconferencing units and trained their cameras on the ceiling or floor of the clinic. Some sessions were dominated by a single speaker. Others had long silences with no one clearly at the helm. Our overall impression was that use of videoconferencing is still in an experimental phase and that the technology's culture of use could benefit from constructive leadership by those who possess the skills to weave an engaging presentation.

In terms of presentation content, the local experts leading the discussions tended to enforce linkages between clinical and community-based systems. We observed presenters explaining clinical concepts, such as diabetes-related nutrition or diagnosis of depression, in terms of community-based paradigms. These paradigms connected patient behaviours to social outcomes and described patient states of health and wellness in terms of mind, body and spirit. Many of the presenters also drew on historical forces, such as residential schooling or the decline of traditional lifestyles ('living on the land'), in their analyses of the current state of health care and community well-being.

We had a much harder time interpreting the positions of the audience members in most of the sessions we viewed. Rarely did members of the audience join in the presentation or offer feedback. Administrators at KO Tribal Council told us that this apparent lack of audience participation may in some measure be explained by norms held in the communities. Indeed, respondents from our preliminary encounter group told us that First Nations in the Zone do not like to interrupt speakers, and take time to ponder new information before offering feedback. They also told us that as videoconferencing is relatively new in many of the First Nations, less experienced para-professionals may feel unfamiliar and shy when they see the possibility of taking centre stage on the video display.

To further explore the CTC and community health workers' perceptions of the Zone's emerging e-health curriculum we undertook a series of focus groups with members of the five KOTH/M First Nations that had originally joined our study. In total, 35 individual participants, CTCs, community health representatives and community health workers participated in five focus groups[14] to discuss their use of ICTs on the job. What we learned was that, overall, internet/web-based information systems do appear to contribute to their roles, but more needs to be done to enable effective use.

Of the 35 participants, the majority (more than 80 per cent) indicated that they search the internet to learn about health issues specific to their work and/or of concern to their community. In terms of the frequency of searching, 25 per cent of the majority indicated searching less than once a week but more than once a month, and 25 per cent indicated searching less than once a month but more than once every six months. The rest indicated searching less than once a month. When asked about the search engines or specific websites that they most frequently use to find information to support their health care work, 80 per cent indicated google.com as their first choice. Other responses included: yahoo.com, 'any search engine is good enough', K-Net.ca, NAN health (a regional First Nations portal), and webmd.com. Almost 90 per cent of respondents also noted the weekly use of email to contact peers for programme-related support, including access to work-related health information; 74 per cent indicated using instant messaging, but only about a quarter of that group indicated using it for work communications.

When asked whether they search for work-related health information that is specifically classified as First Nations, 50 per cent indicated no, some with the condition that they wanted information specific to a particular health issue; 25 per cent indicated yes, and 25 per cent indicated ambivalence. When asked about the kinds of health information topics they look for, the respondents unanimously mentioned health issues in their communities (asthma, diabetes, speech pathology, foetal alcohol syndrome, eczema, and so on) as well as broader issues pertaining to community well-being (child care and discipline, family separation, family violence, drugs and alcohol, and mind/body/spirit therapies).

From the focus groups it became clear that KOTH/M videoconferencing, and particularly education sessions, provided the greatest portion of the respondents' ICT-mediated health information. When asked about other sources of health information, top responses were that the health clinic provided a comprehensive source of health information where books and pamphlets from various regional health organizations could be ordered, and in-person advice could be sought from peers and clinicians. Moreover when asked about the media sources they depend on to disseminate health information, the majority of respondents mentioned community radio or community cable television (if available), posters in the health clinic or Band Office, and word of mouth as primary strategies, possibly followed up by email campaigns or a local website if technical support was available. It is evident from these responses that the local health clinics are the primary information spaces for people to meet and discuss community health issues.

Conclusion

Our research in the Sioux Lookout Zone, in which we have brought together data from a number of sources, indicates that First Nations health care para-professionals, community health workers, community health representatives and community telehealth coordinators straddle a dual system which contains clinical and community-based health care components. Though they act as mediators between the different components, they perceive themselves primarily as representatives of community-based health care, entrusted by the First Nations (and FNIHB Health Canada) to support patients undergoing clinical care, address deeper spiritual and emotional needs, and reinforce linkages between community well-being and personal health. Through the work of these para-professionals, health clinics in the First Nations are not simply nursing stations for visiting clinicians and points of clinical contact for patients. They are important places for community-based health care.

The emergence of e-health policy through telemedicine and other ICT-based systems within KOTH/M simultaneously affirms and challenges the clinicians' and para-professionals' roles in the health clinics. As KOTH/M moves beyond its pilot phase, the prevailing sustainability model attributed to its future growth and operations stipulates a dominant role for telemedicine based on a narrow conception of e-health: the reduction of non-emergency, medical-related travel. We acknowledge that it is important to consider efficiency in remote health care contexts, but we are wary of sustainability models that focus too narrowly on the clinical aspects of First Nations health care. Such models risk alienating patients and para-professionals who measure the value of health care systems in terms of their impact on community well-being, as well as individual patient health. They may also risk overtaxing clinical staff if complementary support systems are not encouraged to develop in these communities.

Under the KOTH/M pilot project, CTCs emerged as community mediators specifically tasked to support telemedicine and other emerging First

Nations e-health systems. At this stage in the lifecycle of KOTH/M, CTCs appear to grapple with their identities in the dualistic health care system, and clearly assign priority to education and training opportunities, suggesting that capacity-building in this group of workers should be a priority for policy-makers.

Under current conditions, CTCs appear to identify more readily with community health care and less readily with its clinical systems counterpart. If this observation is correct, CTCs may be at risk of becoming confined to a too narrow conception of e-health to the detriment of a fuller appreciation of the ways in which ICTs can and will likely change health care in their communities. Without a fuller appreciation of e-health they may find themselves less able to support patients.

We do not mean to suggest that community-based health care paradigms, as enacted by community health workers and represented by the KOTH/M education sessions we observed, should not contribute in some part to CTCs' education and work roles, just as we do not mean to suggest that telemedicine is not a valuable clinical service in remote First Nations health care. However, there does not appear to be a consistent career path for individuals who may wish to provide the necessary services to help First Nations health administrators and health clinics adopt, adapt and implement emerging (federal and provincial) e-health systems. Moreover, FNIHB Health Canada, the federal department that could logically help shape such a career path, appears too focused on the implementation of telemedicine and less attentive to the needs of the community systems that can make implementation successful as well as possible. What we perceive is a collective need that resonates with a number of existing investors and support organizations at the federal and provincial levels. Within FNIHB Health Canada alone there appear to be multiple funding programmes for clinical and community-based initiatives, each with its own directives to become e-health compatible. Similar programmes exist at the provincial level.

Through e-health, both clinical professionals and community paraprofessionals will increasingly be called on to utilize ICTs in their work with patients in the remote First Nations. They will surely come to require more local support to shape and manage these ICTs and could therefore benefit from a professional e-health mediator. Ideally, such a mediator would help them choose and implement the right applications, whether videoconferencing, online information searches or other computer-mediated activities; and help local stakeholders to integrate e-health with community policy.

Reassigning resources from the existing health care system to create this new mediator role is not the solution. Clinical professionals and community para-professionals in the Zone have full workloads in caring for community members, and placing more technical requirements on their shoulders without appropriate support may diminish patients' quality of care. Moreover, systems change implies deeper cultural change. How health care practitioners on either side of, and in between, the dual health care systems 'consume' ICTs reflects their professional and para-professional identities. Framed by such identities the value of ICTs can become too narrowly focused on particular themes, such as telemedicine and averted travel. For the average community health worker, doctor or nurse, ICTs are applications that augment health care practices and are not sources of core competencies with which to identify their practice.

New 'cultural circuits', new ways of seeing the value in ICT applications, need to be grafted onto the existing health care context if a robust e-health system is to take root in the First Nations. KOTH/M's creation of the community telehealth coordinator (CTC) role is a policy move in the right direction, but to establish pathways to e-health in the circumstances we have observed, a major concerted effort is required to invest in and promote a robust health informatics curriculum.

Our research in the Zone indicates that, in mid-2007, the state of education and preparedness among community members remained a major challenge to establishing an appropriate cultural context for a local e-health mediator role. Clearly, education and career development need consideration in any model of sustainable e-health development in the Zone. It may be that investments in these areas will primarily produce benefits in the long run; however, without substantially more strategic investment in community capacity now, the e-health systems that will emerge are unlikely to achieve the efficiencies and positive outcomes that policy-makers and community members desire.

Notes

1. To use the Indian Act of 1876 as an historical point of reference.
2. More than one First Nation in the Zone re-emerged from the drowning wake of hydroelectric dams feeding industry and urban growth to the South.
3. The first Crown-sponsored residential schools for native children emerged around 1883.

4. That obligation is based on treaties signed between representatives of the First Nations and the Crown over 100 years ago, which continue to define the First Nations' territorial boundaries and rights to public services such as health care and education.

5. This is not to suggest that the federal and provincial bureaucracies of Aboriginal health care act as a single policy unit. What we describe is their common ideological belief in the value of e-health (and the targets of efficiency, access and quality of care) which leads them to collaborate on the development of infrastructure and the implementation of policy change.

6. KO officially represents and works for five First Nations in the Zone: Deer Lake, Fort Severn, Keewaywin, North Spirit Lake, and Poplar Hill. Through the K-Net initiative KO has come to work with all 24 First Nations including their representative Tribal Councils and agencies. To mitigate intertribal disputes, K-Net applications such as KO Telemedicine are governed by committees consisting of board members from across the First Nations and relevant Zone organizations.

7. The name change has been attributed to conflicts with another telehealth programme in Ontario that provides health information to patients through a toll-free telephone number. We wonder if the choice of KO Telemedicine as opposed to KO E-health does not also indicate an attempt to narrow community policy.

8. This is an abbreviated description which does not take into account the enhanced security features of the connection and the layers of scheduling that takes place at KOTH/M and K-Net Services to mitigate disruptions when and where community bandwidth is scarce.

9. A telemedicine consult may typically consume between a third and a half of a remote Zone community's available bandwidth given the current configuration of the network in 2007. QoS is therefore a necessity.

10. Currently, FNIHB pays CAD $800/month or almost a third of K-Net Services' total monthly connectivity charge per community.

11. These community concerns were specifically raised at a series of provincial conferences on Aboriginal telehealth organized by KO Tribal Council and the Chiefs of Ontario in 2006.

12. If telemedicine is to become a standard medical practice, physicians will require clear guidelines for deciding how long network sessions should last, and unsalaried physicians will need to know how much they should charge the provincial medical system for different kinds of sessions, including visitations with patients, immediate family, and follow-ups with other clinicians.

13. A random sample of 30 education sessions was reviewed by the team. We did not undertake a systematic content analysis, but were watching to acquire a general impression of the experience.

14. Five groups of seven participants each.

9

'We're all out there busting our guts, trying to do the best that we can for our people': Health Intermediaries in Australian Indigenous Communities

Lyn Simpson, Michelle Hall and Susan Leggett

Indigenous people[1] continue to be amongst the most disadvantaged people in Queensland and their health continues to lag behind that of other Queenslanders: on average, Indigenous Queenslanders die 20 years earlier than their non-Indigenous counterparts and experience a much higher burden of disease, including chronic diseases, injury and many infectious diseases. Concerted efforts should be continued across sectors to improve the socio-economic status of Indigenous Queenslanders, promote healthy living, deliver existing and new models of health service within the principle of self-determination and community control, and increase the representation of indigenous people in health professions.

(Forster, 2005: xvi)

In a research project called 'Partnering with Community Information Intermediaries to Deliver Health Information in Rural, Regional and Remote Australia',[2] we investigated health information seeking and sharing in rural and remote communities in the state of Queensland. During the project we were particularly drawn to the experiences of Aboriginal Health Workers (AHWs) who, as health information intermediaries in their communities, were charged with addressing the circumstances of extreme disadvantage faced by Indigenous Australians as described above. We interviewed 33 health workers (Aboriginal and white) who are involved in Indigenous health services[3] about their roles in mediating between the orthodox, Western medical system and Indigenous

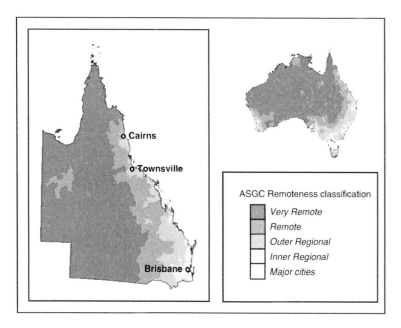

Figure 9.1 ASGC Remoteness Classification, Queensland, Australia
Source: Public Health Information Development Unit (2001).

ways of understanding health and about the impact of their work on the overall health and well-being of their communities.

Many of the AHWs who took part in the study serve remote regions of the country (see Figure 9.1). The most distant of their worksites is more than 2,000 kilometres from Queensland's state capital, Brisbane, and more than 700 kilometres from other cities in the region centres, Cairns and Townsville. The majority of the AHWs we interviewed operate from government-supported Community Health centres which provide community health, child health and sexual health services. A small number were employed by non-governmental organizations (NGOs), in advocacy or support roles.

In this chapter we investigate the intermediary role of AHWs[4] in the context of du Gay et al.'s (1997) circuit of culture framework. This allows us to investigate the interplay of a government-imposed *representation* of AHWs as a culturally appropriate response to the Indigenous health crisis and the resulting *regulation*, where government policy that insists 'only on fundamental and revolutionary social change' (Syme, in Hunter et al., 2003: S52), but often fails to offer guidelines for effective and practical implementation, thereby perpetuating the health inequities suffered by Indigenous Australians. The 'culturally appropriate' representation discussed here is a value-laden term that does not reflect the multiple identity roles conferred on or adopted by AHWs and hence restricts opportunities for 'modest but practical' responses at the community level (Syme, in Hunter et al., 2003: S52). Our research indicates that paying attention to these multiple identity roles reveals the potential value of overlooked tools and technology as practical responses that may assist AHWs to more effectively carry out their work as health intermediaries.

Indigenous health and the western medical system: the need for intermediaries

The AHW is an important element in the complex relationship between Australia's often crisis-focused health system, which is founded on the scientific 'medical model' of hospitals and doctors, and the health beliefs and requirements of the Indigenous peoples it purports to serve. Western medicine's focus on the individual is greatly at odds with the beliefs of Aboriginal and Torres Strait Islander peoples, for whom health is 'not just the physical well being of an individual but is the social, emotional and cultural well being of the whole community' (National Health Strategy Working Party, 1989: x). As in Canada (see Fiser and Luke, this volume), for Australia's Indigenous people, health involves a close relationship with the physical environment and a sense of personal connection with the total well-being of the community (Burden, 1994; Trudgen, 2000). These relationships have been significantly eroded by European settlement, contributing to a poor health status for many Australian Indigenous people (Burden, 1994; National Health Strategy Working Party, 1989; Tregenza and Abbott, 1995; Trudgen, 2000).

Like hard-to-reach populations elsewhere, Indigenous Australians suffer significant health inequalities in comparison with the general population. This has been linked to systemic discrimination (Aboriginal and Torres Strait Islander Social Justice Commissioner, 2005: 13) associated with the lack of equitable provision of infrastructure and services to Indigenous Australians. Distance exaggerates this inequity. Although Aboriginal people comprise only 2.4 per cent of the entire population of Australia, they make up 25 per cent of the remote and very remote population (National Rural Health Alliance, 2006) and suffer disproportionately from disadvantages, such as limited supplies of fresh food, poor road and telecommunications provision, limited education and employment opportunities, inadequate housing and reduced access to health care and public health infrastructure.

Because they live in remote regions, Indigenous people often have limited access to health care providers, many of whom are available on a temporary or visiting basis only and offer treatment on a fly-in/fly-out schedule which may vary from once a fortnight to once a year, or even longer. Gaps in medical service are often filled by government Community Health centres or Aboriginal Community Controlled Health Services which operate as interfaces between hospitals (often located in a distant regional centre) and the Indigenous population and also provide local facilities for various visiting allied health professionals and NGOs. The turnover of medical staff in Community Health centres, remote hospitals and visiting services is high; many nurses, for example, are employed on contracts of just 6–12 weeks' duration. High staff turnover, as well as a reduced and inconsistent presence of health care providers, reinforce a disjuncture between the formal health system and the Indigenous community, providing limited opportunities for health staff to understand the Indigenous community and its specific requirements. This affects all stakeholders: hospital staff and visiting medical workers often lack cultural awareness and communication skills to engage meaningfully with their Indigenous patients; patients often lack English-language skills and (Western) health literacy to comprehend and manage their medical situation; and patients' families and communities are often unable to draw attention to or have addressed other non-medical contributors to poor health outcomes. In this climate, the role of an intermediary becomes vital; a constant local 'health' presence is needed who can appreciate both the needs and expectations of the Indigenous patient and community, as well as the capacity of the formal health system to respond. In rural and remote areas of Queensland it is the AHWs living in the community who most often fill this role. AHWs coordinate and support visiting health professionals and contract staff by acting as their local representatives in the community. They also monitor and tend to the health status of community members between visits and work to 'smooth over' gaps in communication and cultural understandings, as this AHW notes:

> Acknowledging what the health workers . . . the roles, because a lot of people don't [have an] understanding of what the roles are because there's nothing structural or – what do you call it? – defined, because we are multi-skilled people and we are in many ways. . . . We're also not just a health worker, we're an alcohol and drug worker, we're a mental health worker, we're sexual health workers, it's right across the

board, and we don't have that paperwork to say that we are specialized
in that area, but at least we got the . . . and you have to because there
is no one else for them to turn to.

As information intermediaries, AHWs are relied on heavily by their
communities, resulting in various complications and pressures, as this
Visiting Specialist noted:

That's their expected role from the community to them, for them
to spread that information about what services are around, and the
community get quite irritated and agitated if that doesn't happen.
If they find out later that a service was in and they haven't heard
about it, the health workers will often cop a bit of flak about that
because very much it's their job to do that and if they happen to be
away or they're not around, it just, sometimes it just falls down.

These complexities, along with the multiple skills required of the
AHW role, captured our attention and led us to explore how AHWs
who work in rural and remote communities contribute to their communities' health outcomes. Given the current emphasis on information
and communication technology (ICT) as a potential solution to health
issues in rural and remote areas, we were also keen to understand the
AHWs' attitudes about the value of ICTs in supporting their health
intermediary work.

The representation and regulation of AHWs: 'culturally appropriate' intermediaries

The role of the Aboriginal community health intermediary is positioned
in government policy as a bridge between the delivery processes of the
Western medical system and the needs and beliefs of Indigenous people.
This cultural brokerage role is seen as fundamental in enabling 'services
to be provided in forms, structures, settings and languages with which
the local Aboriginal and Torres Strait Islander communities can identify
and which they will utilize' (Queensland Health, 1994: 11). In the following section we draw on the notion of representation (du Gay et al., 1997)
to explore how the intermediary role is portrayed in government policy
as a 'culturally appropriate' response to the Indigenous health crisis and
how this representation (and a limited understanding of the role's true
nature) influences the regulatory framework governing AHWs' work.

The involvement of Indigenous people in their own health care is seen
by many to be vital to successful health outcomes (Australian Indigenous

Doctors Association, 2005; Productivity Commission, 2005; National Rural Health Alliance, 2006). Indigenous people are more likely to access health care and be satisfied with its delivery when an Indigenous practitioner or health worker is involved (Standing Committee on Aboriginal and Torres Strait Islander Health, 2002; National Aboriginal and Torres Strait Islander Health Council, 2003; Australian Medical Association, 2004). However, the employment of Indigenous people in the Australian health system lags significantly behind that in other countries such as New Zealand, Canada and the United States, with Aboriginal and Torres Strait Islander people making up only 0.9 per cent of the health workforce (Australian Indigenous Doctors Association, 2005; Productivity Commission, 2005). AHWs (who generally have little or no medical training) are often the only Indigenous health contacts available to Indigenous patients. This places considerable responsibility on them to be 'culturally appropriate' intermediaries to represent their Indigenous culture and the needs of their Indigenous patients and to negotiate the formal health system. Within government policy documents, however, there is little exploration of exactly what being 'culturally appropriate' entails, or how health workers should operate (whether they are Indigenous or not) (see, e.g., National Health Strategy Working Party, 1989; Standing Committee on Aboriginal and Torres Strait Islander Health, 2002; National Aboriginal and Torres Strait Islander Health Council, 2003; Aboriginal and Torres Strait Islander Health Workforce Working Group, 2004; Social Health Reference Group, 2004; Australian Health Ministers' Advisory Council, 2006). Instead, cultural appropriateness is used as an indistinct principle to describe a provision requirement, such as 'culturally appropriate health services', 'culturally appropriate environs' and 'culturally appropriate data collection methods' (National Aboriginal and Torres Strait Islander Health Council, 2003: 6, 23, 27). Generally, government policy positions the idea of cultural appropriateness in the work of Aboriginal health intermediaries as *what* needs to be done, but is vague on *how* this works in practice.

Despite continued calls for a clear definition of the role of the AHW (Tregenza and Abbott, 1995; Curtin Indigenous Research Centre, 2002), a need endorsed in the *Aboriginal and Torres Strait Island Workforce Strategic Framework* (Standing Committee on Aboriginal and Torres Strait Islander Health, 2002), a nationally agreed job description that incorporates a core competencies framework and provides guidelines for actively supporting workers in these roles, is yet to be formalized. Without a clear definition or understanding of what their responsibilities entail, AHWs and their non-Indigenous colleagues struggle to manage the weight of government and community expectations. Clarified role requirements and improved regulation and recognition of AHWs are needed (Standing Committee on Aboriginal and Torres Strait Islander Health, 2002) but, in the absence of such clarity, a jack of all trades approach dominates.

For AHWs and health service providers in Indigenous communities, the lack of clarity over the role of the AHW can result in a failure to recognize or respect the cultural knowledge of these workers. In the following passage, an AHW in our study expresses concern over non-Indigenous health workers' willingness to engage with AHWs:

> One of the things is they come in with this information given to them before they even get to [very remote town], so they have this picture already painted and ... I think that they need to be aware that the health worker should be the first point of contact and the local community council, you know, and stuff like. Be respectful in those sort of – and I mean, that's the basic tool.

While government policy documents suggest that AHWs will assume responsibility for the delivery of culturally appropriate health care, these same policies give little attention to the importance and complexities inherent in the role. The positioning of AHWs as 'culturally appropriate' intermediaries is a value-laden ideal, with little in the way of practical frameworks to support it.

Reproducing representations through regulation: the problem of implementation

The representation of 'cultural appropriateness' in Indigenous health is reproduced through regulatory policies guiding AHW recruitment, training, resourcing, remuneration, case management and interaction with colleagues and superiors. However, the lack of clarity about the practical aspects of this representation means that effective implementation is thwarted, resulting in a vicious cycle of unclear representations and inappropriate policy responses. While governments appear to have accepted the need to address Indigenous health holistically, 'they have not engineered their health programs consistent with this understanding nor considered the impact of their broader policy and program approach on Aboriginal and Torres Strait Islander health' (Aboriginal and Torres Strait Islander Social Justice Commissioner, 2005: 11). As a result, AHWs often find themselves undervalued, under-trained, under-resourced and under-supported (Hunter, 2003; Curtin Indigenous Research Centre,

2002; Forster, 2005). In response, numerous reports commissioned by Federal and State governments, the Australian Medical Association and the Australian Indigenous Doctors Association investigate Indigenous health discrepancies in general, and the role of the AHW in addressing them. The resulting documents (Queensland Health, 1999; Curtin Indigenous Research Centre, 2002; Standing Committee on Aboriginal and Torres Strait Islander Health, 2002; National Aboriginal and Torres Strait Islander Health Council, 2003; Access Economics, 2004; Australian Medical Association, 2004, 2005; Social Health Reference Group, 2004; Australian Indigenous Doctors Association, 2005; Productivity Commission, 2005; Australian Health Ministers' Advisory Council 2006; National Rural Health Alliance, 2006) make similar recommendations regarding the purposes of the AHW role and offer similar practical solutions to barriers limiting the role's effectiveness. For instance, the *Aboriginal and Torres Strait Islander Health Workforce National Strategic Framework* (Standing Committee on Aboriginal and Torres Strait Islander Health, 2002), which was endorsed by all States and the Federal government, identifies a number of principles to encourage, maintain and support Indigenous people working in health services. Yet, as is evident in a recent review of the Queensland health system (Forster, 2005) and statements by the Aboriginal and Torres Strait Islander Social Justice Commissioner (2005), and reinforced by our research participants, translating policy into practice is a complex process which is complicated by the unclear, value-laden and often one-dimensional representation of the AHW as a culturally appropriate health service broker.

The failure to translate policy into practice is illustrated by the following examples of issues that AHWs and service providers face in their attempts to reconcile the gap between government representation and regulation of their role and its practical requirements. An NGO team leader speaks of the complexities of training and remuneration in very remote areas where staffing levels are already unsatisfactory:

We went through the process of looking at the pay scales of Indigenous health workers ... we determined one rate of pay for this person, to be told that we couldn't really employ this person and let her work with the other people in [very remote town] because she would be getting more money ... we were a bit gob-smacked about all of that ... it was like when we opened this can of worms with the health workers when we were talking about that. I guess it showed their dissatisfaction with the level they were being paid at. ... What happens is that if the workers are trained, because there's no positions for them at other levels, as trained workers, they would then have to do the work being paid at the less rate.

Balancing regulatory requirements with reality is also illustrated by this comment about delivering health education campaigns and the actual responsiveness of the Indigenous community:

> So we have to do things in Murri[5] time and Murri place and I think that's where we let ourselves down – the message is not getting through to the Indigenous people because we're not picking the right times, the right days, or we're rushing it. We have to rush it to meet deadlines because the bureaucratic people are saying, 'I want this done in three months'. And it's a very good programme but, you know, the number of people who came and attended meetings, even the stakeholders' meeting was poorly attended.
>
> (Director of Nursing)

The challenge of implementing programmes and services for Indigenous communities appears to stem in part from the value-laden nature of cultural appropriateness and is reinforced in government policy frameworks in which there are no clear guidelines about how to carry out the requirements of AHW roles. It is only in non-policy documents, sometimes from Indigenous organizations, that these requirements have been explored in detail. Here, the responsibilities and benefits of AHWs as culturally appropriate intermediaries are understood to include enabling a better flow of personal information resulting from understanding the kinship system, interpreting Western medical terms for Indigenous contexts, acting as mentors and role models for Indigenous children and as leaders and advocates for the community, and building capacity for economic and social engagement (Australian Indigenous Doctors Association, 2005; Productivity Commission, 2005).

In government policy documents AHWs are described as health care workers who assist 'in arranging, coordinating and providing health care' (Department of Education, Science and Training, 2004: 19) and address the cultural gap between Western and Indigenous approaches to health. Within their own communities, however, AHWs are not just one more type of health care worker. Instead, they are always expected to be available, as mediators between Western and multiple Indigenous cultures, as translators and adapters of information and support resources, and as managers of health services in their communities. Varying expectations of AHWs by different stakeholders means that, within the restrictions of their service roles, AHWs must balance the demands of their employer (the formal health system) with those of the community.

'I'm a jack of all trades': flexible intermediaries

To be effective, AHWs need to be flexible in their delivery of health information and care. As an Aboriginal school liaison officer explained:

> I'll use any opportunity – the football training in the afternoon – if something's happened at school and I've got notes or I need to see a parent, I know they're going to be down there and I do the thing down there.

AHWs see the reluctance of other health workers to engage communities in this way as problematic:

> The [mental health] team here needs to loosen up the reins...needs to get out, and go down the riverbed. Go up town. You know what I mean? They need to get out in the community!

For AHWs, it is not just important to provide support, but also to provide it in a way that best suits Indigenous peoples' needs. As the following comments from AHWs suggest, this open, flexible approach is an essential requirement for working successfully in Indigenous communities that generally do not function on a Western time schedule:

> It's hard, it's a big job, I mean it's every day, it doesn't just stop during the day, it's after hours, it's just continuous stuff...it's not just for myself as team leader but all the other health workers here as well, when they socialize, even at home, it's just continuous information given to them...you're always on the ball.
>
> This is a small community and they know where you live too, so they come around to your house!

The AHWs who participated in our study spoke of delivering AIDS education around campfires at night, assisting with dialysis on river banks, taking immunization clinics to the sports field and using street kids to spread personal hygiene messages through their social networks. According to the AHWs, such unconventional methods of service delivery are frowned on by health service bureaucracies. Yet, being prepared to operate outside Western health delivery modes and tailoring help to clients' needs is a fundamental element of AHW practice. Despite promises of

ground-up primary health care provision, metropolitan-based governments appear to lack sensitivity to the local conditions of rural and
remote communities and their implications for AHW intermediaries, or
at least appear unable to account for them in their planning for the delivery of health services (Aboriginal and Torres Strait Islander Social Justice
Commissioner, 2005). As a result, the realities of AHWs' work are not
factored into staffing profiles and AHWs continue to provide services,
on a constant basis, with limited support and resources.

AHWs are considered fundamental to Indigenous health care delivery
because their understanding of their own culture is not easily obtained by
white people. As the following comment by a visiting specialist worker
suggests, such understanding requires multiple identities, including the
ability to negotiate across Western systems of health and government
and to communicate with the Indigenous community:

> We couldn't do it without them. We seriously couldn't do anything
> that we do without the [Aboriginal] health workers, they're our ears
> and our eyes.

Because of the infrequent and sporadic contact between visiting health
service providers and the members of rural and remote communities,
these providers have few opportunities to establish strong networks or
develop trusting relationships with community members. An Aboriginal
health worker commented:

> We still have the movement of agency staff, staff just come and go,
> once they build a relationship, that relationship, they feel confidence
> in coming in and talking to that person, but then that person gets
> up and goes and they don't sort of use, they hate sort of repeating
> or coming back and finding different faces and stuff... they build the
> confidence in coming in and once they find out the person has gone
> they sort of just, they just don't come in.

Visiting health workers have little opportunity to gain a sense of what
is culturally appropriate in Indigenous communities or to build strong
relationships. A visiting school nurse remarked:

> There was so much talk of 'You have to make it culturally appropriate'.
> Everyone uses that term, but nobody tells you what that is! So
> you have to fully ask, 'What do you mean by that?'... I did a
> survey, walked around the community for a full week, going to
> people's houses, going to the women's shelter, council, justice groups,

shop – just wherever I'd call in and just showing them, 'This is what we would like to do'.... So, asking elders and locals if they thought that [particular] issues should be brought into the school.

AHWs generally use community and family networks to distribute and gather information, relying chiefly on face-to-face contact. Although labour-intensive and requiring an ongoing presence in the community, such approaches are regarded by AHWs to be appropriate given the low levels of literacy, lack of telephone infrastructure and an Indigenous cultural preference for face-to-face communication. However, cultural appropriateness is very locally specific; Aboriginal and Torres Strait Islander peoples are not a single 'nationality', and practices and behaviours that are acceptable to one tribal group, or gender within that tribal group, may not be so for others (Tregenza and Abbott, 1995; Trudgen, 2000). Such differences affect the transferability of resources in and between communities, where certain behaviours, although Indigenous, may be culturally inappropriate for specific groups. Aboriginal Community Health team leaders seek to address this issue by employing, where possible, male and female AHWs from different tribal groups.

'It's too white': multilingual intermediaries

Another important role of AHWs is that of translator. AHWs mediate between the written language of the Western medical system and Indigenous understandings of health to ensure that health information is acceptable and useful for a particular audience. Traditionally based in oral cultures, members of Australian Indigenous groups often have low levels of literacy in English, and may speak one or more of the 200 Indigenous languages still in use in Australia. Health information is often presented in English, using medical terminology or Western scientific understandings that may be difficult for people (both Indigenous and non-Indigenous) to understand, which is complicated by a reliance on written text. During our interviews with AHWs, translating such information was an important theme of their intermediary work:

We'll get a white man's resources and then we alter it to ours – to make it more appropriate.... You would have a white man's brochure...[and] then we would turn round and do either PowerPoint or overheads or pictures and alter the wording and everything so it was appropriate, culturally appropriate and not offensive, depending on the type of people.

Doctors and nurses often rely on AHWs to interpret medical prognoses for Indigenous patients. AHWs sit in on appointments or visit patients afterwards to clarify details. This translation role frequently extends beyond health matters with the result that AHWs may provide support far in excess of their paid roles:

> Like, I deal with whatever the problems are. They'll come to me and then I'll just – just say it's legal. I'd refer them to Legal Aid for something or if they just want me to read something to them that they don't understand, well I'll read it to them. It'll be from child health right up until the elders, so it deals with a lot of things. Everything!

Some AHWs do not have the necessary skills in English to interpret Western medical language to members of their community, nor can they explain an Aboriginal person's response or understanding of a health situation to medical staff (Trudgen, 2000; see also Tregenza and Abbott, 1995). Communication can be further complicated by the presence of overseas-trained health staff (often appointed in rural and remote locations) who speak English as a second language. As a result, and despite AHW involvement, medical providers and Indigenous patients sometimes struggle to understand each other (Trudgen, 2000; Hunter, 2004).

'It's like fighting a battle every day': intermediary burn-out

The challenges involved in the many roles required of AHWs contribute to a high rate of burn-out. A school liaison officer explained:

> Sometimes... I'll hide in the car! I've done that... read a book... so I can just have a couple of minutes.

As noted earlier, an understanding of the reality of the AHWs' status as an ever-present source of information and support is not always evident in the documents and policies that proclaim the value of 'culturally appropriate' services. As one AHW commented:

> I mean, most of our line managers think it's just being a team leader and just being a health worker... with the health workers here, the local people and stuff, it's just 24/7, and people don't sort of realize that.

Often, AHWs do not receive the resources, training or support they need in a form that is either practical or 'culturally appropriate' for their own needs:

> *AHW*: And Queensland Health will turn around and tell you that there is a phone number that we can call ... Apparently, it's great for white people! ...
> *AHW*: Yeah, but you won't catch a Murri ringing up some stranger.

Another AHW described the frustration of dealing with departmental bureaucracy and the apparent lack of understanding of conditions on the ground as 'fighting a battle every day'.

Technology: a 'modest but practical' tool for enabling 'culturally appropriate' health care

Du Gay et al.'s (1997) circuit of culture provides a useful way to illustrate the complex interplay between representation, regulation and identity in the AHW's role. What appears to be a lack of understanding about 'cultural appropriateness' and the many identities required of AHWs means that governments regulating the role often overlook alternative means of supporting their work. This is particularly apparent with respect to technology. The remote location of many Indigenous communities means that health workers often suffer from a lack of access to both 'old' and 'new' ICTs. When telephone networks are unreliable, computer and internet connections are in short supply, and vehicles may not only be old but are shared by a number of visiting health workers, then opportunities for peer interaction and access to information are limited. In recognizing the importance of a 'culturally appropriate' approach to Indigenous health care, government policy makers seem to have discounted technology as a tool to support the AHWs' responsibilities.

ICTs are recognized by governments as having a significant role to play in addressing some of the disadvantages faced by residents of rural and remote communities (National Health Information Management Advisory Council, 2001; National Rural Health Policy Sub-committee and National Rural Health Alliance, 2002) and are an assumed necessity for city-based workers. Despite statements that it is 'foolish and inefficient' to expect workers to function without them (Access Economics, 2004: 21), AHWs' access to these technologies is often restricted by poor infrastructure, lack of computers and by intranet access-only policies for some employees. In the documents discussed previously, only non-government publications emphasize the importance of ICTs, both for locally-based training and to assist in the provision of health care (Curtin Indigenous Research Centre, 2002; Access Economics, 2004; Australian Medical Association, 2004).

The policy focus in which Indigenous peoples are represented as requiring a 'culturally appropriate' approach to health service delivery appears to have blinkered governments to the opportunities that ICTs can provide. Although acknowledging that Indigenous people are often affected by the 'digital divide', government policy indicates little attention to the potential for ICTs to provide under-resourced AHWs with more timely access to information, easier means to manipulate information into culturally appropriate forms, or the ability to network and share culturally relevant information with other AHWs located in rural and remote areas. Policy makers have also overlooked successful outcomes from previous exploratory work about videoconferencing, teleradiology, touch screens and Indigenous language translation that have demonstrated the acceptance and usefulness of the technologies for some Indigenous communities (Department of Communications, Information Technology and the Arts, 1999; Hunter et al., 2003; Australian Flexible Learning Network, 2004).

As exemplars of what might be called 'innovation by necessity', AHWs often find inventive uses for whatever technologies are available to them in ways that align with the Indigenous preference for face-to-face communication and visual representation. For example, videoconferencing facilities were used by Indigenous families to maintain contact with relatives who were transferred to hospitals in urban centres (although the intended use of such facilities was to support medical specialists to perform remote consultations). Several AHWs also mentioned the value of the internet for finding and sharing resources with other AHWS or technologies such as PowerPoint for adapting Health Department resources to make them more relevant to local needs. As the following comments suggest, while these technologies are seen by many AHWs as ways to improve access to and alter health information to create localized information materials, most of them lack sufficient access to computers and the internet for such options to be viable, resulting in frustration and additional work:

Aboriginal liaison officer (ALO): You've got access to the computers in the [hospital] kitchen. But sometimes you don't get a chance to get in the kitchen, you know, dining room I meant.

AHW: Yeah, they are always busy. When you go, the doctors are always on them.

ALO: I think internet, again you need that access, whereas you go into the kitchen, into the staff dining room at the hospital, there's only two computers. But those two computers aren't always available. I went in there at 9 o'clock one night.

Conclusion

Applying the concepts of representation, regulation and identity from the circuit of culture (du Gay et al., 1997) to the health intermediary activity of AHWs highlights the gap between the multiple identities required of these workers in practice and their representation in government policy. The disconnection between policy representations and practical identities results in an under-appreciated, poorly supported and under-resourced workforce. While certain regulatory problems are an unavoidable outcome of the costs of health care delivery in remote environments, others may be avoidable, such as through the reasonable provision of technological resources and training, which have the potential to enhance the effectiveness of AHWs' work,

The representation of the AHW role as a 'culturally appropriate' means of addressing the Indigenous health crisis has validity. Only Indigenous people employed in this role can truly understand the contributions of historical, tribal, community and environmental factors to Indigenous health and well-being. Yet, without clearly defined roles and responsibilities for AHWs, as well as practical and meaningful pathways for training and advancement, the importance of their knowledge is degraded and its value becomes abstract. It was clear from our conversations with AHWs that many feel undervalued and under-supported, especially with regard to the role they play in bridging the cultural gap between Western and Indigenous understandings of health. Yet they bear the principal responsibility for addressing the considerable health inequities faced by Indigenous Australians. Simple measures such as the provision of internet access and training could enhance the effectiveness of AHWs in a number of their roles and serve as a significant, tangible acknowledgement of their important contributions.

Notes

1. Australia's Indigenous population comprises both 'mainland' Aboriginal peoples and Torres Strait Islander peoples.

2. The project was funded by the Social Sciences and Humanities Research Council of Canada as part of the Action for Health research programme.
3. We gratefully acknowledge the time, assistance and generosity of the Aboriginal health workers who assisted us in this research. The quotes used in the title of this chapter and in some of the sub-headings come from interviews with these people.
4. People in these roles may be of Aboriginal or Torres Strait Islander origin.
5. 'Murri' is the term used by some Queensland Aboriginal people to refer to themselves.

10
Helpers, Gatekeepers and the Well-Intentioned: The Mixed Blessings of HIV/AIDS Info(r)mediation in Rural Canada

Roma Harris, Tiffany Veinot, Leslie Bella, Irving Rootman and Judith Krajnak

In Canada, an estimated 58,000 people live with HIV/AIDS, with approximately 2,300–4,500 new infections occurring each year (Boulos et al., 2006). Although HIV/AIDS has primarily affected men who have sex with men and injection drug users, an increasing number of women and Aboriginal people are becoming infected (Public Health Agency of Canada, 2006). In recent years, combination drug therapies have revolutionized HIV/AIDS treatment and reduced AIDS-associated morbidity and mortality (Schanzer, 2003; Palella et al., 2006). Unfortunately, however, these therapies do not cure HIV and the demanding requirements of treatment regimes, drug side-effects and potential co-infections mean that people living with HIV/AIDS (PHAs) face considerable challenges (Canadian AIDS Treatment Information Exchange, 2003). As a result, access to accurate, up-to-date treatment information is an essential resource for PHAs and their care-givers, as they make health decisions and provide HIV-related support. Information about HIV transmission is also important for the general public, as individuals make decisions about risk-related behaviours (Johnson et al., 2003).

Information about HIV/AIDS is not always easily accessible, especially for people living in rural and remote areas. In Canada, for example, the limited availability of health care providers in rural settings can be a significant barrier to information access, as is rural dwellers' reluctance to use the services of local AIDS Service Organizations (ASOs) (Health Canada, 2000). As a result, rural residents may have limited local routes to reliable HIV/AIDS information and PHAs must often travel a long way to receive specialized care (Health Canada, 2000). Information accessibility problems can also affect rural health care providers. In the United States, for example, rural physicians may have little relevant training or experience with HIV/AIDS and limited specialty back-up to support their treatment of those with the disease (Reif et al., 2005).

The informal exchange of health-related information is an important health support process, especially where access to formal health care services and professional providers is limited. To explore how information related to HIV/AIDS is exchanged in rural areas and the impact of the information exchange process on community members we conducted interviews with more than 100 participants in three rural regions of Canada as part of a larger research programme, the Rural HIV/AIDS Information Networks Study. Participants were asked about their experiences with HIV/AIDS and how they locate, use and share HIV/AIDS information. Of particular interest were the interpersonal networks used to exchange HIV/AIDS information and the impact of the internet on this process. Rather unexpectedly, the interviews revealed some interesting observations about the exchange of 'misinformation' about HIV/AIDS, which we define as false, misleading or medically unsubstantiated information. In this chapter we examine how such misinformation is located, expressed and shared, describe the impact on community members when false or questionable information about HIV/AIDS is exchanged, and discuss how PHAs, their friends and family members and their health care providers 'mediate' or intervene to correct misunderstandings about the disease.

Relying on du Gay and Hall's circuit of culture (Hall, 1996; du Gay et al., 1997; see also Wyatt, Harris and Wathen, this volume) to frame our analysis, we are able to explore the 'production' of misinformation, as individuals adopt and pass on messages in which 'representations' of HIV/AIDS are embedded, as well as how the internet facilitates the transmission of misinformation from one unsubstantiated source to another. We also describe the various impacts when misinformation is 'consumed' and examine the roles of those who counter misinformation by creating competing discourses, constructing and reconstructing the social identities of both the disease and of those living with it. Because HIV/AIDS is a disease with implications extending beyond those who are infected, misunderstandings about its origin and transmission instil fear, even among those not directly affected. As a result, PHAs may be understandably reluctant to disclose their status in communities where there is little knowledge of HIV/AIDS or where people openly express negative attitudes about the disease. In such settings, stereotypes about PHAs and

mistaken assumptions about HIV/AIDS are less likely to be openly challenged or subject to the same level of interrogation that might occur
in more open-minded communities where the disease can be discussed
more freely. In small towns or sparsely populated regions in which privacy is limited and stigmatization of the disease is high, information about
the disease may be driven underground, to be altered, distorted and move
unchallenged through informal networks (Williamson, 1998).

As with other serious and incurable illnesses, HIV/AIDS is a disease
that can inspire production of information of dubious quality, such
as medically unsubstantiated rumours about 'cures' and treatments, or
conspiracy theories about its origin. Transmission of this type of misinformation is facilitated by the internet, where it can be passed quickly
from one unsubstantiated source to another. While misinformation does
not necessarily originate in rural areas, given the limited formal health
care services in many rural locations, few local health specialists may
be available to counteract it. In this context, the process of information
'regulation' (or its lack), a component of Hall's circuit of culture, is also
relevant.

HIV/AIDS misinformation and its producers

Many of the participants in our study described personal experiences with HIV/AIDS misinformation exchange, or misinfo(r)mediation.
Although the sources of the misinformation varied, its content was fairly
consistent, falling roughly into three categories: information that challenges the severity or local existence of the disease; mistaken notions
about how the disease is transmitted; and unsubstantiated claims about
treatments or cures. We describe these categories of misinformation
below, often using the participants' own words.

Disease denial

Living in a place where members of the general public have little knowledge of HIV/AIDS or believe it does not affect anyone around them can
be a challenge for PHAs and those who support them. A number of interviewees reported that their neighbours seemed unaware of the existence
of the disease locally or held stereotyped views about those it affects:

> I just think that this community is very closed-minded and very closed
> off, and I think that a lot of the times if you were to poll this town . . .
> people would say, 'It doesn't affect me, it has nothing to do with me'.
> (friend/family member)

> People don't believe it exists in our community. It's a denial thing.
>
> (health care provider)

> When I was in elementary school, we were taught that AIDS was a gay,
> black man's disease ... not a lot of people in the area were informed
> on this.
>
> (friend/family member)

This representation of HIV/AIDS as 'other', or belonging to groups outside the community, may contribute to the typical observation among
participants that the disease is not perceived as a problem in their community. Others in the community may be generally aware of the disease,
but play down its severity. Several health service providers commented
that young people in particular may believe mistakenly that advances in
HIV/AIDS treatment mean that the illness is no longer life-threatening.
One health service provider said:

> You sometimes hear comments like, 'Well, you know, the reason
> they're not putting as much money into HIV and AIDS these days
> is because we're not seeing new infections anymore', or 'The drugs do
> such a good job controlling the disease now it's not a big deal if you
> get HIV anymore'. I find those sorts of comments, especially coming
> from young people, very, very concerning.

As a service provider in another region observed: '[o]ne of the biggest
ones I remember hearing was ... that um, "Oh well it's OK, you know, if
I get AIDS or HIV, then I'll just take a cocktail," and I'm like, thinking,
oh dear Lord.'
   At the extreme end of the continuum of denial are those who believe
that HIV/AIDS does not really exist – one PHA told the interviewer that
the media over-dramatize the disease and fail to report cases of individuals who recover because HIV/AIDS is a money-maker for health care
providers and pharmaceutical companies. He bases his doubts about
what physicians say on his personal experience:

> I have a deep doubt that this HIV exists. I have been thinking that
> this might not be a real thing, was something invented.... I know
> people that have been living with this disease for 30 years and they
> don't have any sign and they don't have any symptoms, so if that's
> something that's going to kill them then they should be affecting
> them in one or in another way. But when you don't feel anything in

your body, you don't feel absolutely nothing, it's just that the doctor is telling you that you have such and such thing, but in fact the doctor has been telling me that my body is responding much better than he thought it will be, because my viral load's gone up and up and up, I am almost in 1200 CD4 – normal person is only 500 – so I'm … normal person. So, is this a true virus or maybe just an invention? … I don't believe what the doctor is telling me because the doctor is not God. And even though he has the papers that came from the lab, they can still commit some mistakes.

The internet plays an important role in supporting and promoting this man's extreme beliefs. He shares his ideas extensively with others online and has found sources on the web that bolster his views, such as AIDS denial literature, which he describes as having been published by scientists.

Transmission myths

Some of the most common misunderstandings about HIV/AIDS have to do with the ways in which the disease is spread from one person to another. As one of the service providers remarked: 'There's so much misinformation out there. People still think that they can get it from mosquitoes.'

Many of the interviewees had encountered examples of transmission 'myths'. In the following passage, a family member of a PHA who died in 1995 explained:

Maybe for a year after he died they were all … getting tested. I even got tested. People were concerned too because they breathed the same air as him, and they touched him … people were really worried, you know, if they could get this disease just talking to him.

Regrettably, although more than a decade has passed, these myths persist. As one recently diagnosed PHA said:

Often people still are so afraid that they really do feel like … they can, um, be infected by kissing or sharing food, like people are just basically not wanting to touch or get near or close to you, or even breathe the same air.

In the experience of one family member, men often believe that exposure to HIV is only a problem for homosexual men, whereas the women she knows fear other means of transmission: 'Women are concerned about eating off the same dishes as someone who's positive, or having their baby around somebody who's positive, like, you know, like babies are going to absorb it through the skin or something.' When such views prevail, a helpful PHA putting his hands in the dishwater is seen as putting others at risk: 'He was helping at a church dinner and doing dishes, and she just, it was terrible, "you shouldn't be doing dishes," you know. "What if he cut himself and there would be blood in the water?" '

Misunderstandings about HIV transmission are not restricted to lay people. One respected provider of complementary and alternative medicine told our interviewer about a 'cover-up' of the ease of transmission of HIV, and that it could 'in fact' be transmitted by tears. Additionally, during the interviews repeated references were made to local health care providers who were poorly educated about HIV/AIDS, gave incorrect information or were afraid of being infected by their patients. For instance, one of the health care providers in the study described a health care provider in an urban hospital serving many rural PHAs who did not want them to have access to the staff washroom. In another example, a nurse who had cared for her son as he was dying of AIDS in the mid-1990s, reported that one of her colleagues told her that she ought not to return to work until she had been tested for the disease for fear that she would infect her patients.

Other interviews revealed beliefs that deny transmission realities, such as a conviction that love or religious faith can prevent infection. One woman who is HIV-positive told our interviewer that her husband (who had not tested positive) refused to use condoms during sex in order to demonstrate his love for her. Another woman explained that she and her husband decided not to practise safe sex, even though she is HIV-positive and he is not, because of their religious faith:

> We just believe God has put us together and that if he's put us together, nothing's going to happen. . . . I'm sure people think that's, you know, stupid thinking, but we just believe that if God has put us together nothing bad is going to happen that's going to pull us apart and that's faith.

Longing for a cure

People who live with an incurable illness and those who love them are understandably interested in any information which hints at a better outcome. So, it was not entirely surprising that some PHAs reported they had heard of or read about existing or imminent cures. As one man explained,

'There's the new pill coming out ... that you can take with your regular medication, and within six months the virus has gone out of your system.' Another PHA believed a friend who told him that the government has a cure for HIV that they have not yet released. As the following passage suggests, misunderstanding about HIV treatment, combined with a desire for a cure, can draw people to accept misinformation:

> We had one family member who was talking to another family member of another PHA who said her child was cured. ... So they wanted to know ... is this a possibility? ... It's just misinformation around the viral loads. The person had undetectable viral loads ... and the Mom said the child didn't have it anymore, so this kind of brought a little bit of hope ... people will grasp at anything ... in that situation and, you know, they certainly can't be faulted for that.
>
> (health care provider)

Several interviewees trust alternative treatments to prevent HIV disease progression, although most of these treatments are unsupported by medical evidence. For example, a family member of a PHA told the interviewer about her belief in herbal remedies:

> The medical community all say the same thing. And, um, I've never really agreed with the medical community on a lot of things because I've seen people get better and or prevent things ... my experience has been when you start reading about some of these herbs that they can do amazing things and I've seen them do amazing things.
> *Interviewer*: So what has been the answer in terms of what you've learned in terms of treating HIV through alternative methods?
> *Respondent*: One thing that there's some herbs that they tell people not to take. Specifically, um, milk thistle. Well, their livers are inundated with drugs and become toxic and they expand. I mean, it usually isn't the HIV virus that kills them, it's some opportunistic infection or, um, a side-effect from a drug or whatever. ... I knew two people, they were a couple, two guys, and one took all the medications and he was very sick and couldn't do anything. The other one did it all naturally and you wouldn't have known that man was sick. He worked, he did everything.

Providers of alternative medicine may also purport to offer alternatives to medical treatments for HIV disease and may encourage vulnerable individuals to believe in these alternatives. For example, a sister of one of the PHAs told us that her homeopath was 'positive' he could effect a cure if only her family member would pursue the treatment. Some PHAs also described the involvement of friends and relatives in network marketing of health products they tried to sell to them with a promise of 'immune boosting' or other vague benefits.

While those with business interests may pressure PHAs to consider alternative or unusual treatments, friends and family members can also play pivotal roles in promoting unsubstantiated remedies. While well intended, such information is not always welcome. As one PHA explained:

> It's kind of like getting a bad gift, you know, that you didn't want.... I know that they want to be helpful but ... I try and tell them that you're really not going to find anything new. If you found it, I already know.

The desire for a cure combined with unmonitored and excessive use of alternative or supplemental health products can be dangerous. A PHA commented:

> [S]ome people ... they love all these vitamins. They read and read and read on vitamins and next thing you know they have hoards of vitamins because it's going to do this to their immune system or it's going to do something else to the immune system and so they have, you know, 10 or 15 bottles of vitamins, but they're taking another 10 or 15 bottles of other pills to treat depression, to treat whatever, liver disease, Hepatitis C, it's all in combination with their HIV, and then they get their HIV meds and the next thing you know they're hospitalized because they're full of toxicity.

Health care providers, too, expressed concern about the potential dangers of untested remedies to which misinformed PHAs may turn. One physician remarked, 'People can't really be putting unknown substances like that into their bodies without running the risk of it interfering with some of the medications they may be taking. They actually might be making themselves worse.'

Misinfo(r)mediaries

Most of those interviewed try to avoid passing on information of questionable value and, as we will discuss later, many have worked hard in their local communities to challenge misinformation and misunderstandings about HIV/AIDS. However, a few of the study participants had been involved in 'production' activities that might best be described as misinfo(r)mediating. When transmitting dubious clinical advice, promoting unproven products or just passing on information of questionable value, the internet is an important vehicle that permits info(r)mediators to connect to a potentially broad audience while remaining anonymous and remote from any consequences. In the following passage, a non-medically trained PHA, quoted above, whose ideas denying the existence of the disease are suggestive of conspiracy theory, describes how he uses the internet to give clinical advice to others:

> A guy was dying eight months ago, in the hospital, in the United States. A person called me through the internet and I ... communicated with his mother, and ... later on with him, by telephone. [I] told him to leave the hospital if he didn't want to die.... He believed in us better than the doctors, so we advised him to take juice, rice juice, you know ... the diarrhoea would stop. So we advised him to do that first and he did it.... [and I told him] about other medicine, natural medicine. He weighed 40 kg when he was in the hospital. Eight months later he is weighing now 79 kg.
>
> *Interviewer*: OK. So, so you ... gave advice to other people to help them.
>
> *Respondent*: I don't want to do that, but people ask me for that so I'll do it.... I just give them some advice on how to take the natural medication, what kind of exercise they should do, what kind of lifestyle they should start taking ...
>
> *Interviewer*: OK, so these are the three people that you talk to on the web?
>
> *Respondent*: Oh no, that's hundreds of people.

This example illustrates the ease with which a dedicated layperson can take on a health (mis)info(r)mediary role and use the internet to reach – and possibly influence – a great number of people.

Identity and disease representation: misinfo(r)mediation and isolation

While misinformation may endanger PHAs who accept false or unsupported treatment information, misinfo(r)mediation can also have a significant negative impact on the social interactions of those who are affected by HIV/AIDS. A lack of information or the exchange of misinformation about the disease can be damaging and painful for PHAs, as well as their friends and family members. Many interviewees described the fear, hurt and silencing they had experienced as a result of ignorance, mistaken assumptions and negative stereotypes about the disease:

> Um, when I first contracted the disease ... the majority of my friends were straight, and they all gave me lots of misinformation about the disease, that I was totally infectious, everything that I touched would be disease-ridden ... I worried, um, that I would infect my family. I didn't know. I knew very little about HIV when I got HIV, so I, I thought that it was passed through body fluid so I thought if I cried and my tears got into, introduced to a member of my family onto their face and they wiped it away or it got into the mouth, I worried that I would infect them.
>
> (PHA)

> There's a lot of people who just don't know a thing about the disease, and probably do not realize that there's someone that is currently in their life that is living with it in silence because of them and people like them.
>
> (health care provider)

HIV/AIDS is often perceived as a disease that is exclusive to gay men. This can be problematic for PHAs, especially in communities where religious organizations play a prominent role in opinion-shaping. For faith-based groups that regard homosexuality as a sin, PHAs may be represented as reaping the 'wages of sin', as having brought the disease upon themselves. Such representations can be upsetting for PHAs and their families. As one PHA put it, 'At that point a lot of the churches felt that this was a punishment from God, so the question was "What did you do that you're being punished for?"' Another commented, 'I don't need Jerry Falwell [American televangelist] telling me I'm going to hell.'

Ignorance about disease transmission can also position PHAs as people to be avoided or feared and can cause rifts between PHAs and others in their family and community, generating feelings of hurt, isolation and rejection:

> His sister was ... always saying some crazy things about bleaching everything. You had to bleach all the dishes and ... it really hurt his feelings.
>
> (friend/family member)

Like I have one friend who had invited me over once. She knew before she invited me over that I was HIV-positive.... She invited me over for lunch and I forgot something and went back and she was putting my dishes in the garbage, that I had used for lunch.... And I've never been back to her house and she avoids me like the plague.

(PHA)

When I contracted HIV, half my friends didn't want to be my friends anymore. These were straight people that had irrational fears and literally felt they were going to catch the disease if they touched me.

(PHA)

Misinformation about HIV/AIDS not only disrupts relationships between friends and family members, but can stigmatize entire communities. When a number of women became infected in one small rural community, not only did the Red Cross stop bringing the blood donor clinic to town but, as a health care provider explained:

We were getting a lot of negative media attention. We had a community that was kind of devastated in more than one way. We had youth that couldn't go to sports events because they couldn't get billeted because we were the HIV/AIDS capital of the world.

Counter-info(r)mediating

In our study, we found that rural-dwelling PHAs are often significant local sources of accurate and up-to-date information about HIV/AIDS. Sometimes, because they may be among the very few informed people in their communities, PHAs feel they must assume an active educational role to counter stereotypes and challenge misunderstandings. Some do so by taking advantage of 'teachable moments' arising in conversation, for example:

I was doing a job one time and this kid was working there, he was, I don't know, 19, 18 years old. This was about six months after I was diagnosed. And one day, he's going ... 'Yeah, people with AIDS. That's just God's way of killing all the fucking scum on the Earth.' And I said, 'Oh, you really think that, eh?' And he said, 'Aw, yeah, there's no doubt about it, fucking gays'.... And I said, 'You know I've got AIDS, eh?' And he went, 'Oh yeah, whatever!' ... And I said, 'I'm not kidding.' His mouth just dropped and his whole story changed [*laughs*]. . . . I just let him go and go and go and then finally I told him.

Friends and family members of PHAs can also be important advocates working to increase tolerance and correct misunderstandings about the disease:

> Once in a while I'll give a 10-minute commercial on it [*laughs*] ... I will stand up if I heard anybody say anything negative. I would certainly ... try to have them understand that possibly they're not quite as informed as they should be. . . . 'Well wait a minute; well, I don't think you know quite all the figures there', you know?
> *Interviewer*: And what sparks those discussions? How does it get started?
> *Respondent*: Um ... some guy that ... doesn't know what they're talking about. How do I explain that? Ignorance. . . . I don't, certainly don't jump all over him, but I try to make them ... think they're possibly looking at [it] ... not the proper way.

Health care providers also play an important role in correcting misinformation about HIV/AIDS, including intervening when their colleagues are poorly informed (a role not discussed in the practice literatures of the professions described by Bella et al., this volume). Like the friends and family members of PHAs, health service providers must tread carefully and use their diplomatic skills to be effective info(r)mediaries. Several mentioned that they found it effective to challenge transmission myths by describing their personal experiences with PHAs. As a participant from an AIDS service organization explained:

> Um, in most instances it is a request, you know, 'How can I convince, you know, um, my partner that the kids aren't at risk if I come home?' ... The information is that you're not at risk, you know, if you go hug or kiss somebody who's HIV-positive. I have four grandkids who have been in this office and have hugged grandparents who are HIV-positive and when I share that story it probably gives more reassurance than the, the academic information. . . . Because, um, we all kind of know each other in a small community. That has a lot of impact. What you do is a lot more important than what you say.

Health care providers can also counter misinformation acquired from the internet. Although many respondents appreciate the internet as an information source about HIV/AIDS, some noted its troubling potential as a source of misinformation:

> It can help reduce isolation if you can connect with people. Um, and … it also can be a place where people are taken advantage of, um, and where there's inaccurate information that can really make people anxious.
>
> (service provider)

> It's a mixed blessing … because if you get into one of those *fear-mongering* websites, you can be convinced you're dead in six months…. That happens, and people get so terrified because of this doom and gloom and 'God's judgment' and 'white man conspiracy' and all this nonsense that we come out with such a warped view of what HIV is. That they're going to die next week, you know, and it's not good.
>
> (PHA)

Several health care and service providers explained how they intervene when PHAs and others are affected by misinformation obtained from the internet. Using techniques that librarians would call 'bibliographic instruction' or 'user education', they explain to their patients or clients the importance of assessing the trustworthiness and reliability of material located over the internet:

> Upon intake we give them a package with really good sites that they can access that we think are reliable and trustworthy for information. So if a client has brought in something that's sort of hearsay or from the internet, you know, I'll usually get online with them and I'll go and say, 'This is maybe why I wouldn't use this site' um … if I don't feel it's, it's reliable information. And I would try to go to a site and say, you know, 'This is a really good site, we encourage you to use this and this is what they say on this. So, I would, I would probably trust this information more than I would trust this one, you know.' In fact, sometimes I would completely discourage them from access or, you know, following through on whatever the information was that was provided to them…. They could go away again and access a new website, so it's really about giving them the tools to understand what's a good website and what's not, right?
>
> (service provider)

Understanding (mis)info(r)mediation

To varying degrees, the issues we have explored in this chapter involve each of the processes described in the circuit of culture (Hall, 1996; du Gay et al., 1997). With respect to 'consumption' and 'production', for example, it is clear that the methods by which information about HIV/AIDS is obtained and the sources responsible for producing the information have a significant impact on PHAs, their friends and family members, and their health care and service providers. Through the informal exchange processes that occur in small communities, inaccurate and occasionally damaging information passes from one person to another. Those who are better informed may avoid comment, remaining silent to avoid being stigmatized. Although the internet can overcome the constraints of local geography by enabling access to reliable, up-to-date information about this complex disease condition, it can also be used to propagate misinformation. Vendors of 'alternative' products and misguided info(r)mediaries who offer 'cures' or question the severity of the disease can produce misinformation that flows freely through the internet.

Misinfo(r)mediation and resulting misinformation exchange can contribute to the spread of HIV because mistaken beliefs about who is likely to 'catch' the disease or incorrect assumptions about its 'treatability' may create a false sense of security in some who engage in high-risk behaviours. No regulatory framework controls or contains the passage of questionable or potentially harmful information, especially when it is exchanged, or even produced, by laypersons. Community members, no matter how well-intentioned, who pass on unsubstantiated or inaccurate information about transmission or treatment of HIV/AIDS, may put others at risk. However, when such information is exchanged outside the formal health system, there are few limits on how information about the disease can be produced and transmitted, or by whom. In the absence of regulation, and in rural settings that are remote from specialized services, those infected or affected by HIV/AIDS often play a significant role in producing counter-discourses that are more closely aligned with widely accepted biomedical and epidemiological knowledge about the disease.

The social processes of 'identity' and 'representation' are also pertinent to the health information exchanges we have described. The social identity of PHAs and the positioning of their illness as a disease of irresponsibility or 'otherness' is a major subtext in the misinfo(r)mediation process. The interviews clearly revealed the hurt and isolation caused by information exchanges in which victim blaming, stereotypes and transmission myths are reinforced. Such exchanges perpetuate misunderstandings of the disease that, in some instances, cause unnecessary fear, further contributing to the isolation and silencing of those who are infected, affected and in need of support. However, as PHAs and their family members, friends and service providers engage in infomediary work, mobilizing counter-discourses to challenge misinformation, they contribute to the emergence of the new social identity – the 'local AIDS activist'. Those who assume this identity are proud of their public commitment to fighting the disease. Despite the worrisome misinfo(r)mediating practices described in this chapter, it is encouraging to witness the concerted efforts of community members who challenge ignorance and the spread of misinformation. Their use of counter-informing strategies to reduce the impact of misinformation about HIV/AIDS, and to insert new or 'better' information into the community health information exchange process, is a crucial and generally unacknowledged function of both lay and professional health info(r)mediaries who are affected by this disease.

Note

1. The Rural HIV/AIDS Information Networks Study was funded by a grant from the Canadian Institutes of Health Research under the HIV/AIDS Community-Based Research Program. Study regions were located in Newfoundland and in rural regions of Ontario and British Columbia. Data gathering in one of the study regions was also supported by funding from the Social Sciences and Humanities Research Council of Canada, Collaborative Research Initiatives, Initiative on the New Economy, 2003–2008 for the Action for Health project, 'The role of technology in the production, consumption and use of health information: Implications for policy and practice'.

11
Reflections on the Middle Space

Nadine Wathen, Roma Harris and Sally Wyatt

In this book, we have described examples of the actors and relationships in our 'middle space', that amorphous ground between end-users – those 'health-interested' seekers of various kinds of health information and care – and the broad and sometimes murky universe of health information. This final chapter weaves together some of the threads drawn to our attention by the contributors, presents emerging themes regarding the actors and their relationships in this middle space, and considers the implications of these themes for those making policy and practice decisions in health care and health information support. We begin with a discussion of how 'users' of health information are defined and situated, then explore specific aspects of info(r)mediation as they affect end-users, with a particular focus on features of mediators that seem to facilitate or be a barrier to the info(r)mediation process; ending with some implications for policy and practice in the areas of health care and health information services. It should be noted that our focus is not so much on health information itself, but the process of health information mediation and how it varies, depending on such contextual factors as professional role, the presence of information and communication technologies, and various sociotechnical configurations. To this end, the 'circuit of culture' has provided an analytical framework for situating the actors and their interactions within the set of processes that we call 'health info(r)mediation'.

The 'health interested': How health information and help seekers are situated

One interesting theme in the present analysis is how health information seekers are described, discussed and situated. Consistent with the broader health and social science literatures related to this topic, the labels applied to 'end-users' vary quite broadly, even within this book. In an attempt at neutrality *vis-à-vis* both the source and use of information, some authors prefer labels such as 'layperson' or simply 'user'. In contrast, other labels, such as: 'patron', 'client' and 'patient', constitute and, one might argue, restrict the role of the information seeker in terms of the help they seek (see Bella et al., this volume). The terms used to describe end-users reflect nuanced differences in the ways in which info(r)mediation processes occur. More commonly in the recent literature on this topic 'consumer health information' is applied to describe any tool or resource produced for non-professional, health-interested people, and by extension, those who seek and use such resources are called 'consumers'. While touched on in the chapter by Henwood et al., an examination of this particular label and what it invokes (Hibbard and Weeks, 1987; Grace, 1991; Lupton, 1994) is beyond the scope of the present analysis. However we find this term problematic and refer instead to 'health information seekers' to describe the behaviours and needs of people in this context. In cases where these seekers actually do use a technology or information, we refer to them as 'users'.

Related to the issue of labels is the position of the health information seeker with respect to both what is being sought (information in a broad sense, but often also care and support) and the actors mediating the process. Again, in this book, how the user is represented in the information seeking and exchange process depends largely on the nature of the mediation process, the interplay of domains in the 'circuit of culture' and, to some extent, the distance between the information seeker, the information producer and the mediator. For example, Sanders, and Balka and Butt highlight some important aspects of the use of websites as mediators. A key goal of many of the users of the men-for-men websites described by Sanders is increased social proximity, however a feature of these and most websites is 'distance' between the producers of information (in this case both the website sponsors and public health authorities) and those who visit the sites. Similarly, Balka and Butt demonstrate how the language of the BC Health Guide online portal situates visitors as consumers of health information and makes some highly problematic assumptions about the role of online information in 'empowering' users to make better health decisions.

On the other hand, the mediation processes described in several chapters are, at least in their presentation, far more person-centred. This is best exemplified in the two chapters describing the emergence of new roles in the health care system that are designed to bridge cultural divides which have been identified as barriers to appropriate and effective health care. Both Fiser and Luke and Simpson et al. describe the key role played by para-professional Aboriginal health workers in translating the needs of their community members into terms understood by the Western health care system, and, conversely, transforming medical information and procedures into culturally appropriate forms of care. This transformative role best illustrates Latour's (2005) distinction between intermediaries and mediators, as quoted in the opening chapter of this volume. Harris et al. provide a good example of 'high touch' and person-centred information mediation, but in the context described by these authors this may come at the potential cost of accuracy and reliability of the 'facts' being exchanged. As this chapter again demonstrates, the transformative nature of Latour's mediation is neither value-neutral nor always beneficial to the health information seeker.

Somewhere between these 'high(er) tech' and 'high(er) touch' contexts are the examples provided by Bella et al., describing the roles of health and social service professionals as formally constituted in their standards and mandates, and by Henwood et al., describing the public library as a space in which health information seekers have access to resources both online and (ideally) mediated more directly by professional librarians. In both chapters, the information seeker is positioned as a 'service receiver' who is constituted uniformly within professional discourses (with some inter-professional variation).

Another emerging theme is the concept of 'hybrid' sociotechnical configurations either accidentally or explicitly created to address identified gaps between what health information seekers need and what systems can provide. Three such examples, though somewhat different in their emphases, are described by Pennefather and Suhanic, Sanders, and Fiser and Luke. These authors present mediators that explicitly combine an ICT with a human role. In the case of Fiser and Luke, the new role of 'community telehealth coordinator' emerged as a result of the decision to implement telemedicine applications in a remote Aboriginal community. Existing roles that were not technically-oriented (the community health workers and representatives) were not deemed sufficient to address the specific challenges (and opportunities) presented by integration of the technologies and processes parcelled within 'telemedicine' (and later 'telehealth'). The further development of specific web-based tools to support this work is an example of how these hybrid forms can continue to evolve in intended and unintended ways. The discussion of the various bridging functions served by this new role and its supporting tools (regarding technology implementation but also between different conceptualizations of health and health care systems) provides insight into how such processes, which are often consequences of policies decided from afar, might be analysed.

Pennefather and Suhanic also propose a new hybrid configuration that is explicitly tied to a technical product, namely the digitized diagnostic image. By situating the technology as a site for consultation and exchange between human actors (primarily clinicians and patients), their 'narrative diagnostic image' may highlight the best kind of sociotechnical mediator, where the technology is simply a tool to facilitate human engagement.

An interesting set of questions raised in any analysis of processes where improving the experiences of health information seekers in finding and using resources is a stated goal, is how these users are positioned with respect to the information, its producers, and those providing mediation. Are people being 'cared for', 'cared about' or 'cared at'? Are they seen as experts in their own health and illness experiences and their health-related needs? Or, are they constituted as patients or clients who are expected to comply with expert directives? What kind of control and choice do information seekers have in terms of both when and how they gain access to information, and what exactly is retrieved? To what extent is communication (between end-users and information producers and mediators) one-way, with no or limited opportunity for interaction, or two-way (i.e. more interactive and dialogic)? Do information seekers have control over the timing of what they receive? Enhanced interactivity implies synchronous communication between the user and source/mediator; however, for complex or emotionally challenging information, asynchronous communication might sometimes be preferred, as it gives people time to reflect on information they receive. In terms of the examples provided in this book, the answer to most of these questions is: 'It depends ...'

Who and what are the 'go-betweens' and what work do they do?

As will have become evident, health info(r)mediation and info(r)mediators are terms that describe numerous relationships between information sources and health information seekers. Figure 11.1 summarizes our conceptualization of the actors and their positions in the health info(r)mediation process. The types of sources, mediators and seekers' needs all vary widely and, as a result, each part of Figure 11.1 merits deconstruction and analysis. However, we focus our discussion on the

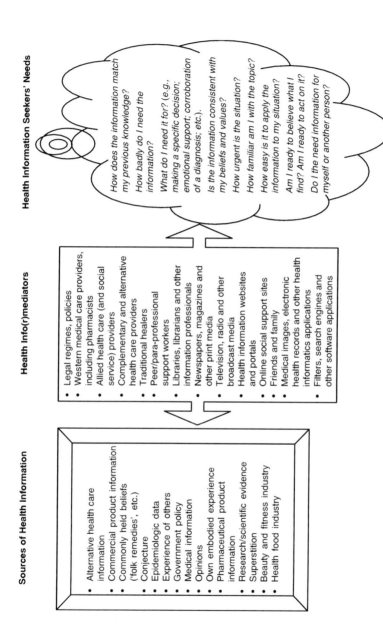

Figure 11.1 Representation of sources and seekers of health information, and types of info(r)mediators

middle, and highlight some of the factors that seem to facilitate or inhibit the ability of health information seekers to get what they need.

A striking feature of the 'middle' (the arrowed box in Figure 11.1) is the breadth of types and roles of mediators. First, and obviously, is the (intentionally simplistic) continuum from 'solely ICT' to 'solely human' or the 'high(er) tech'/'high(er) touch' aspects discussed above. However, even seemingly simple typologies are complex when examined closely. For example, the library setting described by Henwood et al. would seem fairly 'physical' (as opposed to virtual) with an interactive human focus as 'patrons' consult with librarians. However, the policy decisions which influence this health info(r)mediating site, along with expectations regarding the roles of both librarians and technologies (public computer access terminals) in this setting, have complicated that context since, as Henwood et al. describe, the professional role is ceded in large part to the technology (the internet access provided by the terminal) to the extent that the response of library staff to the 'dangers' of the internet in the context of health information is to encourage users to rely on a very limited number of government-sponsored or approved websites. Thus the experience of many library patrons, perhaps contrary to their expectations, may be entirely with an ICT-based mediator – the internet, and whatever health websites they happen to come across.

Another interesting feature of the different types of mediators is their 'visibility' to the health information seeker. This may be related to how 'technological' the mediator is, but not exclusively. Figure 11.2 captures this aspect. On the left one can see that, from the seeker's perspective, other people (in their various formal and informal roles) are highly visible: users will readily be able to identify the mediator and (presumably) be more able to assess the value (however self-defined) of the information provided. On the far right side of Figure 11.2 are examples of the 'invisible' mediators described in this book, in particular the internet content filters discussed by Gibson and Sutherland and the popular internet search engines described by Balka and Butt. We have placed the other types of mediators at different points on the continuum to reflect our interpretation of how users seem to view them.

The methods of info(r)mediation and the levels at which they occur also vary greatly. The chapters highlight that the mediation process occurs between and among: individuals directly (e.g. health information seekers and their clinicians, family members, friends, community health workers); individuals mediated by technology (such as 'narrative' diagnostic images; men seeking men via websites); collectives mediated by technology (health information content produced for communities

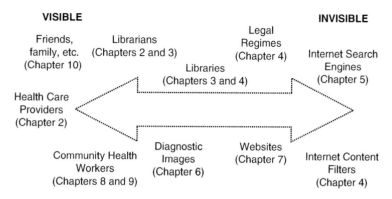

Figure 11.2 Visibility of health info(r)mediators to information seekers

or populations of users and pushed out via the internet), and more traditional means (library collections, mass media); and individuals and systems mediated by human actors (Aboriginal health workers) or technologies (telemedicine applications), or both (community telehealth coordinators).

Similarly, the modes of communication used by mediators vary (as mentioned in the previous section) from synchronous, face-to-face interactions to downloading static (filtered or unfiltered) information from a website. Ideally, the mode and channel of communication will match the health information seekers' needs, skills and context, as described on the right side of Figure 11.1.

It's only getting messier

The health information seeking and mediating processes described in this book are complex as well as time- and resource-intensive. Decisions to allocate resources to specific mediators mean that other mediators, human and otherwise, will not be supported. This situation is unlikely to get easier or cheaper as the amount and variability of health information continues to expand; new and complex diagnostic and other health-related technologies emerge; and citizens are increasingly expected to be 'informed' and 'sensible' decision makers regarding their own health care (Henwood et al., 2003; Nettleton et al., 2005). To understand the forms that might best serve both citizens and health support systems, it is helpful to consider, from the perspective of the health information seeker, the features of health info(r)mediation and info(r)mediators most likely to provide benefit.

What makes a 'good' health info(r)mediator?

From the examples presented in this book, it appears that effective mediators have a number of key characteristics in common. First and foremost, whether they are web-based or human, mediators that are local, interactive and personalized seem to have the greatest chance to be preferred and used by health information seekers – a finding consistent with previous literature in this area (Harris and Dewdney, 1994). This is exemplified by Simpson et al. and by Fiser and Luke in their discussions of the role of Aboriginal health workers whose specific purpose is to 'localize' Western medicine to make it culturally appropriate. This is also evident in the description by Sanders of the emergence of avatars and tailored information for gay men, and by Pennefather and Suhanic in their description of 'personal' diagnostic images.

The chapters that closely examine interactions between individuals, where the complexities of the mediator role are especially evident, highlight several features of these concepts of 'local', 'interactive' and 'personalized' that are of interest. First, info(r)mediation seems to be facilitated when mediators, including health professionals, are part of social networks relevant to the health information seeker; or when they are readily identified by the seeker as being 'like me'. This network link not only conveys a point of access between the mediator and the information seeker, but also the imprimatur of credibility and trust necessary to allow the seeker to make value judgements about the information provided (Wathen and Burkell, 2002).

Second, mediators who are able to be flexible and are willing to work outside of formal structures to gain trust are particularly valued by health information seekers. Conversely, those who are bound by strict role expectations may not be able to serve the diverse needs of those seeking help. The ability to balance the demands of different 'sides' and multiple identities (different health systems and beliefs, and different personal roles of being health workers and Aboriginal community members, for example) is ideal from the health information seeker's perspective. However, this is not always possible, or necessarily desired by those occupying different places in the 'system', including, as Bella et al. show, the mediators themselves. Conversely, too much flexibility, such as that afforded to those without a professional code of conduct or other means to standardize their information-giving, can be just as, or even more, damaging.

This is exemplified in the discussion by Harris et al. of '(mis)information' flow in HIV/AIDS information-sharing in rural areas.

Another facet of flexibility is the ability of mediators to serve different ends – sometimes concurrently. Sanders' description of men-for-men (M4M) websites includes their use by public health officials as a means to promote health information to what is perceived to be a high-risk population. This appropriation of websites to serve public health ends reflects a very different goal from the initial reason for the sites' creation. In fact, in his analysis Sanders describes M4M sites as an emerging 'contested medium'.

Related to this is the issue of how health-seeking individuals or communities may resist efforts to appropriate info(r)mediators and processes for these unintended purposes, a concept related to what Brown and Duguid (2000) call 'gatekeeping'. They argue that not all gatekeepers are 'obtrusive'. However, in the face of too much 'access', people may start actively seeking out their own, preferred kinds of gatekeepers.

Implications for policy and practice

What does this discussion tell us that could be of practical value for those making policy and practice decisions in the provision of health care and health information support? First, it is clear that human actors engaged in mediator roles remain integral to health information seekers' ability to find and use health information. In 1994, Harris and Dewdney described several general 'principles' of information seeking, including: (i) information needs are contextual and arise from the situations in which help-seekers find themselves (see Figure 11.1); (ii) people tend to rely on information that is easily accessible, looking first for advice and information from interpersonal sources, especially those 'like me', and rely on formal or institutional sources as a later or last resort (see also Leydon et al., 2000); and (iii) as confirmed in the latter chapters of this book, most people expect information and help to be delivered within a relationship of care – they want providers to demonstrate concern and provide emotional support, conditions that can be as, or more, important than the actual quality of the information provided (see Wathen and Harris, 2007).

Many of the mediator roles described in this book are performed by human actors who are implicitly or explicitly expected/required to 'educate' or 'inform' those they serve. As Bella et al. describe, this educational role is often not well articulated, as many mediators (often health care professionals) do not receive formal training or ongoing support for this function. One practical recommendation, therefore, is to acknowledge the importance of this work by investing in the types of training and continuing education resources that other aspects of these professional roles receive. Significantly, this will increasingly include training in hardware, software and other ICTs, as well as the ability to critically appraise health information not only for its general value, but also its particular worth to the 'client/patient/patron's' situation and needs. These considerations are especially vital in the context of emerging para-professional roles such as those described by Simpson et al. and Fiser and Luke. The challenges of providing 'culturally appropriate' care and serving as a local 'cultural broker' or 'bridge' are acute for people who perform these roles, often without any training or credentials, in the context of very rural and remote settings, perhaps using new ICTs, and sometimes under confused or contradictory policy directives.

An exciting theme emerging from many of the chapters relates to the novel ways in which new sociotechnical configurations are being shaped to meet the needs of those seeking health information and care. However, these examples are offset by concerns about escalating spending on technological 'solutions' that not only fail to work, but also mean that resources are not available for more traditional, person-to-person approaches. The opportunity costs of implementing ICT-based interventions must be factored into decisions about spending, along with some consideration (to the extent possible) of the unanticipated or 'disruptive' consequences of these programmes. Several chapters highlight both beneficial and potentially harmful results of what can happen when policy decision making is driven by untempered enthusiasm for health informatics applications.

Another practical matter to consider when planning programmes to address the needs of health information seekers is who actually controls the info(r)mediation process. Gibson and Sutherland, in their discussion of internet content filters in public libraries, highlight at least three actors with significant, and often divergent, interests: library boards and administrators concerned *inter alia* about liability; library patrons who expect free access to information in a public library; and software vendors who expect to profit from the sale of their products. Articulating these interests and including various protections when developing programmes and policies is vital to avoid the worst kinds of unintended consequences.

People still matter: In fact they seem to matter more than ever

Effective health info(r)mediation is not likely if human mediators function solely as 'warm experts' (Bakardjieva, 2005) or only possess health knowledge. Rather, effective info(r)mediators combine the ability to convey 'care' with the expertise necessary to assist people in finding (often with the aid of relevant ICTs) and interpreting 'good' health information. As Brown and Duguid (2000: xvi) say, we are increasingly prone to '[i]nformation fetishism ... the superficially plausible idea ... that information and its technologies can unproblematically replace the nuanced relations between people'. This 'obsession' with information and information technologies – what de Mul (1999) has called an 'informationistic worldview' – ignores the underlying relationships between people that allow information to be produced and shared in the first place (Brown and Duguid, 2000).

The strength of this book is that it brings together researchers from a number of disciplines who have conducted their work in a wide variety of settings, often from very different epistemological starting points. Du Gay et al.'s circuit of culture provided a framework for analysing different aspects of the info(r)mediation process. It enabled the contributors to this book to focus on different processes associated with the production, consumption, regulation, identity and representation of health information and those involved in its mediation in order to develop a rich understanding of each of these processes individually and in interaction. The result has been to raise a number of interesting and plausible concepts and issues of both theoretical and practical importance. However, this is only the beginning, and we admit to raising more questions than we have answered. For example, we have focused almost exclusively on the info(r)mediation process from the perspective of the health information seeker, and have implied, in many ways, that the success of the process can only be assessed according to the seeker's self-defined outcomes. Is this the correct way to assess the process? It certainly is not the only way, and more research, including other perspectives, units and levels of analysis with multiple (even conflicting) outcomes, is required.

Similarly, in an attempt to keep the arguments clear, we have presented mainly single mediator roles in the various contexts described. However, the reality is often much more complex, especially in emerging online communities. For example, in Sanders' chapter there are potentially multiple mediators, including the website itself, the health authorities providing certain types of content, and the avatars developed by other users. Which one is most attended to and useful will depend on the user's particular needs of the moment. How do we analyse the various mediators and their interactions with site users individually? Can we and should we?

It is inevitable that these mediator roles will continue to evolve, especially as pressure is applied from producers of new technologies, and from increasingly sophisticated users who expect their mediators to engage with them in new ways. There is already a growing literature on, for example, the challenges of 'shared decision making' between doctors and patients and the stresses placed on this relationship when doctors are confronted with patients who have sought to inform themselves and arrive at the clinic with information printed from the internet (Wald et al., 2007).

The next site for analysis may well be the Web 2.0 world. What is the impact of 'local' yet 'distant' mediators, those 'like me' but whom one has never met? As roles blur between avatars in online worlds and humans in the physical world, how will this influence what we are ready to believe, and from whom? Indeed, how will we constitute the 'spaces' of info(r)mediation, or compare, for example, the public library and Second Life as sites of analysis? What will be the impact of open source platforms that allow collaborative ongoing enhancement of information and tools? And finally, do we have the right metrics and analytical tools to assess and measure the purported benefits (and costs) of health info(r)mediation? There is a lot of work to be done.

In this book we have analysed the middle space between health information seekers and what they seek. While many aspects of the health info(r)mediation process require further research and analysis, a key conclusion emerging from this volume is that to assume that one can take humans out of the middle and replace them with 'clean technological pipelines' is not only naïve but potentially dangerous.

Bibliography

Aboriginal and Torres Strait Islander Health Workforce Working Group (2004) *ATSIHWWG Annual Report 2002–2003: A Report on the Implementation of the Aboriginal and Torres Strait Islander Health Workforce National Strategic Framework.* Canberra, Australian Government Department of Health and Ageing.

Aboriginal and Torres Strait Islander Social Justice Commissioner (2005) *Social Justice Report 2005.* Sydney, Human Rights and Equal Opportunity Commission.

Access Economics (2004) *Indigenous Health Workforce Needs.* Kingston, ACT, Australian Medical Association.

ACIET (Advisory Committee on Information and Emerging Technologies) (2005) *Pan-Canadian Health Information Privacy and Confidentiality Framework.* Ottawa, Health and the Information Highway Division, Health Canada, January. Available online: http://www.hc-sc.gc.ca/hcs-sss/pubs/ehealth-esante/2005-pancanad-priv/index_e.html (accessed 15 October 2007).

Adamson, W. (2002) Sex in the city – What happened at the Minneapolis Public Library. *New Breed Librarian 2*(2): 2–6.

Adelson, N. (2000). *'Being Alive Well': Health and the Politics of Cree Well-Being.* Toronto, University of Toronto Press.

Ahmad, F., Hudak, P. L., Bercovitz, K., Hollenberg, E. and Levinson, W. (2006) Are physicians ready for patients with internet-based health information? *Journal of Medical Internet Research* 8(3): e22.

Alexander, P. (1996) Bathhouses and brothels: Symbolic sites in discourse and practice, *in* Dangerous Bedfellows (eds) *Policing Public Sex: Queer Politics and the Future of AIDS Activism.* Boston, MA, South End Press, pp. 221–50.

Allcock, J. C. (2000) Helping public library patrons find medical information – the reference interview. *Public Library Quarterly* 18: 21–7.

American Civil Liberties Union (16 November 2006) ACLU suit seeks access to lawful information on internet. Press release. Available online: http://www.aclu-wa.org/inthecourts/detail.cfm?id=557 (accessed 27 August 2007).

American Civil Liberties Union v. Gonzales. Civ. Action No. 98–5591 (E.D. Pa. 2007).

American Civil Liberties Union v. Reno. 117 S. Ct. 2329 (1997).

American Dietetic Association (1999) Code of ethics for the profession of dietetics, *Journal of the American Dietetic Association* 99: 109–13.

American Library Association (2000) 12 ways libraries are good for the country, *American Libraries Online.* Available online: http://www.ala.org/ala/alonline/selectedarticles/12wayslibraries.cfm (accessed 27 August 2007).

American Library Association (2007) *FAQ about Libraries, Children and the Internet.* Available online: http://www.ala.org/ala/washoff/WOissues/techinttele/internetsafety/faq.htm#filter(accessed 27 August 2007).

American Nurses Association (ANA) (2001) *Code of Ethics for Nurses with Interpretive Statements.* Available online: http://nursingworld.org/books/tocs/codeofethics.pdf (accessed 13 August 2007).

Anderson, B. (1998) Reflection on practice: Dietician as partner or expert. *Canadian Journal of Dietetic Practice* 59(3): 138–42.

Andreassen, H. K., Bujnowska-Fedak, M. M., Chronaki, C. E., Dumitru, R. C., Pudule, I., Santana, S., Voss, H. and Wynn, R. (2007) European citizens' use of e-health services: A study of seven countries. *BMC Public Health* 7(53): 1–7.

Anon (2005) *Stedman's Medical Dictionary for the Health Professions and Nursing*. Philadelphia, Lipincott Williams and Wilkins.

Archibald, G., Cook, L., Jones, S., Newman, W. and Skrzeszewski, S. (n.d.) *Internet Service in Libraries – A Matter of Trust: A Report for the Canadian Library Association*. Available online: http://www.cla.ca/resources/internetservice.htm (accessed 27 August 2007).

Arnold, B. and Boggs, K. U. (2003) *Interpersonal Relationships: Professional Communication Skills for Nurses*. Toronto: W. B. Saunders.

Auffrey, L. (2006) Nurses to pioneer new frontier: The virtual highway. *The Canadian Nurse* 101(1): 35.

Australian Capital Television Pty Ltd v. The Commonwealth (1992) 177 CLR 106.

Australian Flexible Learning Network (2004) *Computer Animation Sends a Message for Good Health*. Available online: http://pre2005.flexiblelearning.net.au/casestudies/casestudies/marvin.pdf (accessed 21 April 2006).

Australian Health Ministers' Advisory Council (2006) *Aboriginal and Torres Strait Islander Health Performance Framework Report 2006*. Canberra, Australian Health Ministers' Advisory Council.

Australian Indigenous Doctors Association (2005) *Healthy Futures: Defining Best Practice in the Recruitment and Retention of Indigenous Medical Students*. Canberra, Australian Indigenous Doctors Association.

Australian Library and Information Association (2002) *ALIA Statement on Online Content Regulation*. Available online: http://www.alia.org.au/policies/content.regulation.html (accessed 27 August 2007).

Australian Library and Information Association (2006) *Advocacy: Online Content Regulation*. Available online: http://www.alia.org.au/advocacy/internet.access (accessed 27 August 2007).

Australian Library and Information Association (2007a) *Internet Access in Public Libraries 2007 Survey Report*. Available online: http://alia.org.au/advocacy/internet.access/internet.filtering.public.libraries.2007.survey.report.pdf (accessed 27 August 2007).

Australian Library and Information Association (2007b) *Internet Access in Public Libraries 2007*. Kingston, ACT.

Australian Medical Association (2004a) *Healing Hands – Aboriginal and Torres Strait Islander Workforce Requirements*. Kingston, ACT, Australian Medical Association.

Australian Medical Association (2004b) *Position Statement on Aboriginal and Torres Strait Islander Health*. Canberra, Australian Medical Association.

Bakardjieva, M. (2005) *Internet Society: The Internet in Everyday Life*. London, Sage.

Balka, E. (2003) The role of technology in the production, consumption and use of health information. Stage 2 project proposal, submitted to the Social Sciences and Humanities Research Council of Canada, July.

Balka, E. and Butt, A. (2006) *Information Seeking Practices of Seniors, Youth and Parents. ACTION for Health Report 2006–07*. Report prepared for the B.C. Ministry of Health. Burnaby, BC, Simon Fraser University, Assessment of Technology in Context Design Lab.

Bastable, S. B. (1997) *Nurse as Educator: Principles of Teaching and Learning*. Massachusetts, Jones and Bartlett.

Baudrillard, J. (1998) *The Consumer Society: Myths and Structures* (trans. C. Turner). London, Sage.

Beck, U. (1992) *Risk Society: Towards a New Modernity* (trans. M. Ritter). London, Sage.

Bella, L., Macinnis, W., Mitchelmore, V., Morgan, J. and St Croix, H. (2005) Using the internet to promote rural health: Towards capacity development for non-profit health agencies. Sixth Conference of the Canadian Rural Health Research Society, Quebec City, October, 2005.

Berg, M., Schellekens, W. and Bergen, C. (2005) Bridging the quality chasm: Integrating professional and organizational approaches to quality. *International Journal of Quality in Health Care* 17(1): 75–82.

Berger, M., Wagner, T. H. and Baker, L. C. (2005) Internet use and stigmatized illness. *Social Science & Medicine* 61(8): 1824–7.

Berkes, F. (1999) *Sacred Ecology: Traditional Ecological Knowledge and Resource Management*. Philadelphia, Taylor and Francis.

Bérubé, A. (1996) The history of gay bathhouses, *in* Dangerous Bedfellows (eds) *Policing Public Sex: Queer Politics and the Future of AIDS Activism*. Boston, MA, South End Press, pp. 187–220.

Bischoff, W. R. and Kelley, S. J. (1999) 21st century house call: The Internet and the World Wide Web. *Holistic Nursing Practice* 13(4): 42–50.

Blocking Software FAQ (n.d.). Available online: http://www.peacefire.org/info/blocking-software-faq.html (accessed 27 August 2007).

Bolding, G., Davis, M., Sherr, L., Hart, G. and Elford. J. (2004) Use of gay Internet sites and views about online health promotion among men who have sex with men. *AIDS Care* 16(8): 993–1001.

Borman, C. B. and McKenzie P. J. (2005) Trying to help without getting in their faces: Public library staff descriptions of providing consumer health information. *Reference & User Service Quarterly* 45: 133–6 and 140–6.

Boulos, D. Yan, P., Schanzer, D., Remis, R. S. and Archibald, C. P. (2006) Estimates of HIV prevalence and incidence in Canada, 2005. *Canada Communicable Disease Report* 32(15): 165–74.

Bowker, G. and Star, S. L. (1999) *Sorting Things Out: Classification and Its Consequences*. Cambridge, MA, MIT Press.

Bowman, L. A., Adams, M. S. and Christopher, A. (2000). Information sources in pharmacy and pharmaceutical sciences, *in* A. R. Gennaro et al. (eds), *Remington: The Science and Practice of Pharmacy*, Philadelphia, Lipincott, Williams and Wilkins, pp. 60–9.

Braman, S. (2006) *Change in State: Information, Policy and Power*. Cambridge, MA, MIT Press.

Brantes, F. de, Emery, D., Overhage, J., Glaser, J. and Marchibroda, J. (2007) The potential of HIEs as infomediaries. *Journal of Health Information Management* 21(1): 69–75.

Brock, S.C. (1995) Narrative and medical genetics: On ethics and therapeutics. *Qualitative Health Research* 5: 150–68.

Brown, G., Maycock, B. and Burns, S. (2005) Your picture is your bait: Use and meaning of cyberspace among gay men. *Journal of Sex Research* 42(1): 63–73.

Brown, J. S. and Duguid, P. (2000) *The Social Life of Information*. Boston, MA, Harvard Business School Press.

Buchanan, D. (2004) Two models for defining the relationship between theory and practice in nutrition education: Is the scientific method meeting our needs? *Journal for Nutrition Education and Behaviour* 36(1): 146–54.

Bunton, A. and Petersen, R. (1997) Introduction: Foucault's medicine, *in* R. Petersen and A. Bunton (eds) *Foucault, Health and Medicine*. London, Routledge, pp. 1–14.

Burden, J. (1994) Health: A holistic approach, *in* C. Bourke, E. Bourke and B. Edwards (eds) *Aboriginal Australia: An Introductory Reader in Aboriginal Studies*. Brisbane, University of Queensland Press, pp. 157–78.

Bureau of Labor Statistics, US Department of Labor (2007) *Occupational Outlook Handbook, 2006–07 Edition*. Available online: http://www.bls.gov/oco/ocos068.htm (retrieved 13 August 2007).

Burroughs, T. E., Waterman, A. D., Gallagher, T. H. et al. (2007) Patients' concerns about medical errors during hospitalization. *Journal on Quality and Patient Safety* 33(1): 5–14.

Cambrosio, A., Keating, P., Schlich, T. and Weisz, G. (2006) Regulatory objectivity and the generation and management of evidence in medicine. *Social Science & Medicine* 63: 189–99.

Canadian AIDS Treatment Information Exchange (2003) *Many Voices: Report on Stakeholder Consultations*. Toronto, Canadian AIDS Treatment Information Exchange.

Canadian Association of Social Workers (2000) *In Critical Demand: Social Work in Canada, Vol. 1, Final Report*. Available online: http://www.casw-acts.ca (accessed 13 August 2007).

Canadian Association of Social Workers (2005) *Code of Ethics*. Available online: http://www.casw-acts.ca (accessed 13 August 2007).

Canadian Association of Social Workers (2006) *CASW Presents the Social Work Profession*. Available online: http://www.casw-acts.ca/ (accessed 13 August 2007).

Canadian Human Rights Commission (2006) *Anti-harassment Policies for the Workplace: An Employer's Guide*. Available online: http://www.chrc-ccdp.ca/publications/anti_harassment_toc-en.asp#11 (accessed 27 August 2007).

Canadian Library Association (2000) *Statement on Internet Access*. Available online: http://www.cla.ca/about/internet.htm (accessed 27 August 2007).

Canadian Medical Association (2000) *Roles of Physicians and Scope of Medical Practice: Future Prospects and Challenges*. CMA Background Paper (May 2000). Ottawa: CMA. Available online: http://www.cma.ca/multimedia/staticContent/HTML/N0/l2/working_on/futures/roles.pdf (accessed 22 October 2007).

Canadian Pharmacists Association (2004) *Position Statement on Cross-Border Prescription Drug Trade*. Available online: http://www.pharmacists.ca/content/about_cpha/who_we_are/policy_position/policy.cfm?policy_id=1 (accessed 13 August 2007).

Canadian Pharmacists Association (2006) *Strategic Plan 2006–2008*. Available online: http://www.pharmacists.ca/content/about_cpha/who_we_are/strategic_plan/pdf/StrategicPlanENG.pdf (accessed 13 August 2007).

Canadian Pharmacists Association (2007) *CPhA Takes Action: e-Information Products*. Available online: http://www.pharmacists.ca/conent/about_cpha/whats_happening/cpha_in_action/einfo_products.cfm (accessed 13 August 2007).

Caplette, N. (1999) *Aboriginal Women's Health in Canada*. Available online: http://www3.undp.org/ww/women-health1/msg00064.html (accessed 1 January 2007).

Caramella, D. (1996) Teleradiology: State of the art in clinical environment. *European Journal of Radiology* 22(3):197–204.

Carballo-Dieguez, A. and Bauermeister, J. (2004) 'Barebacking': Intentional condomless anal sex in HIV-risk contexts: Reasons for and against it. *Journal of Homosexuality* 47(1): 1–16.

Chan, D., Levine, M., Sellors, J. and Howard, M. (2004) Computer networking to enhance pharmacist physician interaction: A pilot demonstration in community settings. *Canadian Pharmaceutical Journal* 137(8): 26.

Charon, R. (2001) Narrative medicine: A model for empathy, reflection, profession, and trust. *Journal of the American Medical Association* 286: 1897–1902.

Chiasson, M. A., Hirshfield, S., Humberstone, M., DiFilippi, J., Newstein, D., Koblin, B. et al. (2003) The Internet and high-risk sex among men who have sex with men. *10th Conference on Retroviruses and Opportunistic Infections (Oral Abstract 8:37)*. Boston, MA.

Child Internet Protection Act, 114 Stat. 2763A-335 (2002).

Children's Online Protection Act, 47 U.S.C. 231 (1998).

Ciborra, C. U. (2002) *The Labyrinths of Information: Challenging the Wisdom of Systems*. Oxford, Oxford University Press.

Ciborra, C. U. and Andreu, R. (2001) Sharing knowledge across boundaries. *Journal of Information Technology* 16: 73–81.

CIUS (2005) *Canadian Internet Use Survey (Record #4432)* Statistics Canada. Ottawa. Available online: http://www.statcan.ca/cgi-bin/imdb/p2SV.pl?Function=get Survey&SDDS=4432&lang=en&db=IMDB&dbg=f&adm=8&dis=2 (accessed 27 August 2007).

Cole, D. (2006) ACLU sues central Washington libraries. *Columbia Basin Herald Online*. Available online: http://www.columbiabasinherald.com/articles/2006/ 11/20/news/news01.txt (accessed 27 August 2007).

Committee on School Health (2004) Soft drinks in schools: Policy statement. *Pediatrics* 113(1): 152–4.

Connor, E. (2000) Using search engines to locate web resources on women's health, *in* M. S. Wood and J. M. Coggan (eds) *Women's Health on the Internet*. New York, Haworth Press, pp. 47–64.

Coonan, H. (2006) *$116 Million to Protect Australian Families Online*. Press release. Available online: http://www.minister.dcita.gov.au/media/ media_releases/$116.6_million_to_protect_australian_families_online (accessed 27 August 2007).

CRaNHR (2006a) *KO Telehealth/North Network Expansion Project*. Available online: http://www.cranhr.ca/onlrpts.html (accessed 1 January 2007).

CRaNHR (2006b) *KO Telehealth/North Network Expansion Project: Appendix 5*. Available online: http://www.cranhr.ca/onlrpts.html (accessed 1 January 2007).

Crespo, J. (2004) Training the health information seeker: Quality issues in health information web sites. *Library Trends* 53: 360–74.

Criminal Code (Canada), R.S.C., 1985, c. C-46.

CSDecode. (n.d.) Available online: http://www.peacefire.org/censorware/ CYBERsitter/csdecode.html (accessed 27 August 2007).

Curley, A. and Broderick, D. (1985) *Building Library Collections* (6th edn.). Metuchen, NJ, Scarecrow Press.

Curtin Indigenous Research Centre (2002) *Training re-Visions: A National Review of Aboriginal and Torres Strait Islander Health Worker Training*. Perth, Curtin Indigenous Research Centre.

Cushman, M. and Klecun, E. (2005) *How (Can) Non-Users Perceive Usefulness: Bringing in the Digitally Excluded*. London, LSE, The Department of Information Systems.

Davis, F. D., Bagozzi, R. P. and Warshaw, P. R. (1989) Perceived usefulness, perceived ease of use, and user acceptance of information technology. *MIS Quarterly* 13: 319–40.

Davis, M., Hart, G., Bolding, G., Sherr, L. and Elford. J. (2006) Sex and the Internet: Gay men, risk reduction, and serostatus. *Culture, Health & Sexuality* 8(2): 161–74.

Dawkins, R. (1976) *The Selfish Meme*. Oxford, Oxford University Press.

Department of Communications Information Technology and the Arts (1999) *From Telehealth to E-health: The unstoppable rise of E-health*. Canberra: Department of Communications Information Technology and the Arts. Available online: http://archive.dcita.gov.au/1999/09/rise (accessed 30 January 2007).

Department of Education Science and Training (2004) *No Shame Job: A Health Career Information Guide for Indigenous Students*. Canberra, Department of Education Science and Training. Available online: http://www.dest.gov.au/NR/rdonlyres/F7716B29–7542–4605–8745–B6603B1D00E9/668/NoShamebook.pdf (accessed 19 December 2006).

Department of Health (2001) *Involving Patients and the Public in Health Care: A Discussion Document*. London, Department of Health.

Department of Health (2004a) *Better Information, Better Choice, Better Health*. London, Department of Health.

Department of Health (2004b) *Choosing Health: Making Healthy Choices Easier*. London, Department of Health.

Department of Health (2004c) *Improving Chronic Disease Management*. London, Department of Health.

Department of Health (2005) *Supporting People with Long Term Conditions: An NHS and Social Care Model to Support Local Innovation and Intervention*. London, Department of Health.

Dewdney, P., Marshall, J. G., Tiamiyu, M. A. and Tiamiyu, M. (1991) A comparison of legal and health information services in public libraries. *Reference Quarterly* 31: 185–96.

DiMaggio, P., Hargittai, E., Neuman, W. R. and Robinson, J. P. (2004) Social implications of the Internet, *in* H. F. Nissenbaum and M. E. Price (eds) *Academy & the Internet*. New York, Peter Lang.

Donaldson, L. (2003) Expert patients usher a new area of opportunity for the NHS. *British Medical Journal* 326: 1279–80.

Dotinga, R. (2004) Legal battle over chat-room STDs. *Wired News*. Available online: http://www.wired.com/news/medtech/0,1286,62005,00.html (accessed 25 August 2005).

Dunn, E., Conrath, D, Acton H., Higgins, C. and Bain, H. (1980) Telemedicine links patients in Sioux Lookout with doctors in Toronto. *Canadian Medical Association Journal* 122: 484–87.

Dworkin, G. (1989) The concept of autonomy, *in* J. Christman (ed.) *The Inner Citadel: Essays on Individual Autonomy*. New York, Oxford University Press, pp. 3–23.

Ealing Library Service (n.d.) *Free Internet Access*. Available online: http://www.ealing.gov.uk/services/leisure/libraries/internet_access/index.html (accessed 27 August 2007).

Eysenbach, G. and Jadad, A. R. (2001) Evidence-based patient choice and consumer health informatics in the Internet age. *Journal of Medical Internet Research* 3(2): e9.

Eysenbach G. and Kohler, C. (2003) What is the prevalence of health-related searches on the World Wide Web? Qualitative and quantitative analysis of search engine queries on the Internet. *Proceedings of the American Medical Informatics Association Annual Symposium 2003*: 225–9.

Fenton, M. (2004) Accessing the keys to life sustaining treatment. *Nutrition in Clinical Practice* 19: 319–23.

Fernandez-Celemin, L. and Jung, A. (2006) What should be the role of the media in nutrition communication? *British Journal of Nutrition* 96: S86–8.

Finch, L. and Warner, J. (1997) *Dividends: The Value of Public Libraries in Canada* [electronic version]. Toronto, Book and Periodical Council.

First Nations and Inuit Health Branch (2006) *First Nations and Inuit Health*. Health Canada. Available online: http://www.hc-sc.gc.ca/fnih-spni/index_e.html (accessed 1 January 2007).

First Nations and Inuit Health Branch (2007) *First Nations and Inuit Health Program Compendium*. Health Canada. Available online:http://www.hc-sc.gc.ca/fnih-spni/alt_formats/fnihb-dgspni/pdf/pubs/gen/cs-133_compendium_e.pdf (accessed 30 March 2007).

Fiser, A. and Clement, A. (2007) *The K-Net Broadband Deployment Model: How a Community-Based Network Integrates Public, Private and Not-for-Profit Sectors to Support Remote and Under-Served Communities in Ontario*. Information Policy Research Program, Faculty of Information Studies, University of Toronto, May 2007. Available online: http://kmdi.utoronto.ca/broadband/programs/Files/fiser_paper.pdf (accessed 1 June 2007).

Fiser, A., Clement, A. and Walmark, B. (2006) *The K-Net Development Process: A Model for First Nations Broadband Community Networks*. CRACIN Working Paper No.12. Available online: http://www3.fis.utoronto.ca/research/iprp/cracin/publications/workingpapersseries.htm (accessed 1 January 2007).

Flicker, S., Buchan, A., Goldberg, E., McClelland, A., Skinner, H., Smith T. et al. (2006) 'Fun & games': Reaching Canadian HIV-positive youth online. *Sixteenth International AIDS Conference*. Toronto.

Flicker, S., Goldberg, E., Read, S., Veinot, T., McClelland, A., Saulnier, P. et al. (2004) HIV-positive youth's perspectives on the Internet and eHealth. *Journal of Medical Internet Research* 6(3): 77–90.

Forster, P. (2005) *Queensland Health Systems Review*. Brisbane, The Consultancy Bureau and Queensland Government.

Foucault, M. (1972) *The Archaeology of Knowledge* (trans. A.M. Sheridan Smith). London, Tavistock.

Foucault, M. (1980) *Power/Knowledge*, ed.C. Gordon. Brighton, Harvester Wheatsheaf.

Frank, R. and Hargreaves, R. (2003) Clinical biomarkers in drug discovery and development. *Nature Reviews Drug Discovery* 2: 566–80.

Freschette, J. (2005) Cyber-democracy or cyber-hegemony? Exploring the political and economic structures of the internet as an alternate source of information. *Library Trends* 53(4): 555–75.

Gardiner, M. (2006) Diagnosis using search engines. *British Medical Journal* 333: 1131.

Gay, P. du, Hall, S., Janes, L., Mackay, H. and Negus, K. (1997) *Doing Cultural Studies: The Story of the Sony Walkman.* London, Sage.

Giddens, A. (2002) *Runaway World: How Globalization is Reshaping Our Lives.* London, Profile Books.

Gillett, J. (2003) Media activism and Internet use by people with HIV/AIDS. *Sociology of Health and Illness* 25(6): 608–24.

Giustini, D. (2006) How Web 2.0 is changing medicine. *British Medical Journal* 333: 1283–4.

Gortler, J., Berghoff, M., Kayser, G. and Kayser, K. (2006) Grid technology in tissue-based diagnosis: fundamentals and potential developments. *Diagnostic Pathology* 1(23): 1–10.

Grace, V. M. (1991) The marketing of empowerment and the construction of the health consumer: a critique of health promotion. *International Journal of Health Services* 21(2): 329–43.

Graham, R. N. J., Perriss, R. W. and Scarsbrook, A. F. (2005) DICOM demystified: A review of digital file formats and their use in radiological practice. *Clinical Radiology* 60: 1133–40.

Gray, N. J., Klein, J. D., Noyce, P. R., Sesselberg, T. S. and Cantrill, J. A. (2005) Health information-seeking behaviour in adolescence: The place of the Internet. *Social Science & Medicine* 60(7): 1467–78.

Griffiths, F., Green, E. and Tsouroufli, M. (2005) The nature of medical evidence and its inherent uncertainty for the clinical consultation: Qualitative study. *British Medical Journal* 330: 511.

Griffiths, J., King, D. W., Tomer, C., Lynch, T. and Harrington, J. (2004) *Taxpayer Return on Investment in Florida Public Libraries: Summary Report* [electronic version]. Florida, State Library and Archive.

Grossberg, L. (ed.) (1996) On postmodernism and articulation, and interview with Stuart Hall, *in* D. Morley and K. H. Chen (eds) *Stuart Hall: Critical Dialogues in Cultural Studies.* London, Routledge, pp. 131–50.

Gulli, A. and Signorini, A. (2005) The indexable web is more than 11.5 billion pages. *Proceedings of 14th International World Wide Web Conference:* 902–3.

Hagel, J. and Rayport, J. (1997) The coming battle for customer information. *Harvard Business Review* 75(1): 53–5, 58.

Halifax Public Libraries. (n.d.) *Internet Access Policy.* Available online: http://www.halifaxpubliclibraries.ca/policies/internet.html (accessed 27 August 2007).

Halifax Public Library (1997) *Collection Development Policy.* Available online: http://www.halifaxpubliclibraries.ca/policies/collection.html (accessed 27 August 2007).

Hall, S. (1992) The west and the rest, *in* S. Hall and B. Gieben (eds) *Formations of Modernity.* Cambridge, Polity Press/Open University Press, pp. 275–320.

Hall, S. (1997) The work of representation, *in* S. Hall (ed.) *Representation: Cultural Representation and Signifying Practices.* London, Sage/Open University Press, pp. 1–11.

Hall, S. (ed.) (1997) *Representation: Cultural Representations and Signifying Practices.* London, Sage Publications/Open University.

Hammond, M. (2006) *Road to Competency: CHRs and the need for national, competency-based training and credible career paths for Inuit, Métis, and First Nations health and wellness workers.* Kahnawake, QC, NIICHRO. Available online: http://www.niichro.com/2004/pdf/road-to-competency.pdf (accessed 1 January 2007).

Hand, M. (2005) The People's Network: Self–education and empowerment in the public library. *Information, Communication and Society* 8: 368–93.

Hannay, T. (2007) Web 2.0 in Science. *CT Watch Quarterly. August 2007.* Available online: http://www.ctwatch.org/quarterly/ (accessed 15 October 2007).

Hansen, J., Holm, L., Frewer, L., Robinson, P. and Sandoe, P. (2003) Beyond the knowledge deficit: Recent research into lay and expert attitudes to food risks *Appetite* 41: 111–21.

Hanseth, O., Jacucci, E., Grisot, M. and Aanestad, M. (2006) Reflexive standardization: Side effects and complexity in standard making. *MIS Quarterly: Management Information Systems* 30: 563–81.

Hardey, M. (2004) Internet and society: Reconfiguring patients and medical knowledge? *Sciences Sociales et Santé* 22: 21–43.

Harris, R. M. and Dewdney, P. (1994) *Barriers to Information: How Formal Help Systems Fail Battered Women.* Westport, CT, Greenwood.

Harris, R. M. and Wathen, C. N. (2007) 'If my mother was alive I'd probably have called her. Nowadays, I turn to the internet.' Women's search for health information in rural Canada. *Reference & User Services Quarterly* 47(1): 67–79.

Harris, R. M., Wathen, C. N. and Fear, J. (2006) Searching for health information in rural Canada: Where do residents look for health information and what do they do when they find it? *Information Research* 12(1): paper 274. Available online: http://informationr.net/ir/12–1/paper274.html.

Health Canada (2000a) *Blueprint and Tactical Plan for a Pan Canadian Health Infostructure, Federal-Territorial Advisory Committee on Health Infostructure.* Ottawa, Office of Health and the Information Highway.

Health Canada (2000b) *National HIV/AIDS Treatment Information Environmental Scan.* Ottawa, Health Canada.

Health Canada (2005) *Blueprint on Aboriginal Health: A 10–Year Transformative Plan, Prepared for the Meeting of First Ministers and Leaders of National Aboriginal Organizations,* (24–25 November). Health Canada. Available online: http://www.hc-sc.gc.ca/hcs-sss/pubs/care-soins/2005-blueprint-plan-abor-auto/index_e.html (accessed 1 January 2007).

Healthwise (2002) *Healthwise Knowledgebase for Canada Localization and Canadian Medical Review Process.* Available online: http://hwinfo.healthwise.org/docs/DOCUMENT/4137.pdf (accessed 14 February 2007).

Heins, M., Cho, C. and Feldman, A. (2006) *Internet Filters: A Public Policy Report* [Electronic version]. New York, Brennan Center for Justice.

Henderson, J. (2005) Google Scholar: A source for clinicians. *Canadian Medical Association Journal* 172(12): 1549–50.

Henderson, S. and Peterson, A. (2002) *Consuming Health: The Commodification of Health Care*. London, Routledge.

Henwood, F., Wyatt, S., Hart, A. and Smith, J. (2003) 'Ignorance is bliss sometimes': Constraints on the emergence of the informed patient in the changing landscapes of health information. *Sociology of Health and Illness* 25(6): 589–607.

Hibbard, J. H. and Weeks, E. C. (1987) Consumerism in health care: prevalence and predictors. *Medical Care* 25(11): 1019–32.

Hoffman, C., Rice, D. and Sung, H-Y. (1996) Persons with chronic conditions: their prevalence and cost. *Journal of the American Medical Association* 278(3): 1473–9.

Howard, J. P., Jonkers-Schuitema, C. F. and Kyle, U. (1999) The role of nutritional support dietician in Europe. *Clinical Nutrition* 18(6): 379–83.

Human Rights Act 1998 (UK) (1998) c. 42.

Hunter, E. (2003) Staying tuned to developments in Indigenous health: Reflections on a decade of change. *Australian Psychiatry* 11(4): 418–23.

Hunter, E. (2004) Communication and Indigenous health. *Australian Doctor*, 4 June: 35–42.

Hunter, E., Travers, H. and McCulloch, B. (2003) Bridging the information gap: IT and health in indigenous populations. *Australian Psychiatry 11*(Supplement): S51–6.

Ibanez, A. (2004) *CTC Workshop Report*. Sioux Lookout, ON, 17–18 November. KO Telehealth/CRaNHR.

Innis, H. A. (1930) *The Fur Trade in Canada: An Introduction to Canadian Economic History*. New Haven, CT, Yale University Press.

Innis, H. A. (1950) *Empire and Communications*. Oxford, Oxford University Press.

Innis, H. A. (1951) *The Bias of Communication*. Toronto, Toronto University Press.

Introna, L. C. and Nissenbaum, H. (2000) Shaping the web: Why the politics of search engines matters. *The Information Society* 16: 169–85.

Ives, T. J., Paavola, F.G. and DerMarderosian, A. H. (2000) Pharmacists and public health, *in* A. R. Gennaro et al. (eds), *Remington: The Science and Practice of Pharmacy*. Philadelphia, Lippincott, Williams and Wilkins, pp. 47–59.

Jaeger, P. T., McClure, C. R., Bertot, J. C. and Langa, L. A. (2005) CIPA: Decisions, implementation, and impacts. *Public Libraries* 44(2): 105–9.

Johnson, B. T., Carey, M. P., Marsha, K. L., Levin, K. D. and Scott-Sheldon, L. A. (2003) Interventions to reduce sexual risk for the human immunodeficiency virus in adolescents, 1985–2000. *Archives of Pediatrics and Adolescent Medicine* 157(4): 381–8.

Johnson, L. C., McClelland R. W. and Austin, C. D. (2000) The worker, *in* N. E. Sullivan, K. Steinhouse, and B.Gelfand (eds) *Challenges for Social Work Students: Skills, Knowledge and Values*. Toronto, Canadian Scholars Press, 83–116.

Joyce, K. (2005) Appealing images: Magnetic resonance imaging and the production of authoritative knowledge. *Social Studies of Science* 35(3): 437–62.

Kadushin, A. (1995) Interviewing, *in* R. L. Edwards (ed.), *Encyclopaedia of Social Work*. NASW, Washington, DC, 1527–37.

Kalichman, S. C., Eaton, L., Cain, D., Cherry, C., Pope, H. and Kalichman, M. O. (2006) Community-based Internet access for people living with HIV/AIDS: Bridging the digital divide in AIDS care. *Journal of HIV/AIDS & Social Services* 5(1): 21–38.

Karst-Ashman, K. K. and Hull, G. H. (2006) *Understanding Generalist Practice* (4th edn). Belmont, CA, Thomson Higher Education.

Kathleen R. v. City of Livermore, 87 Cal. App. 4th 684 (Cal. App. 1st Dist. 2001).

Kay, S. and Purves, I. N. (1996) Medical records and other stories: A narratological framework. *Methods of Information in Medicine* 35: 72–87.

Kemper, D. W. and Mettler, M. (2002) *Information Therapy. Prescribed Information as a Reimbursable Medical Service*. Boise, ID, Healthwise.

Kendall, P. (2006) SNE refines mission and vision, launches project to develop on-line data base for materials promoting my Pyramid and the 2005 dietary guidelines for Americans. *Journal of Nutrition Education and Behaviour* 38: 1, 4.

Kennedy, M. S. (2005) Preventing STDs in African American and Latina girls: When it comes to condom use, practice is better than information alone. *American Journal of Nursing* 105(8): 22.

Kenyon, A. and Casini, B. P. (2002) *The Public Librarian's Guide to Providing Consumer Health Information*. Chicago, Public Library Association.

Kirmayer, L., Simpson C. and Cargo M. (2003) Healing traditions: Community and mental health promotion with Canadian Aboriginal peoples. *Australasian Psychiatry* 11(Suppl.): 15–23.

Kivits, J. (2004) Researching the 'informed patient': the case of online health information seekers. *Information, Communication & Society* 7: 510–30.

Klausner, J. D., Levine, D. K. and Kent, C. K. (2004) Internet-based site-specific interventions for syphilis prevention among gay and bisexual men. *AIDS Care* 16(6): 964–70.

Klausner, J. D., Wolf, W., Fischer-Ponce, L., Zolt, I. and Katz, M. H. (2000) Tracing a syphilis outbreak through cyberspace. *Journal of the American Medical Association* 284, 447–9.

KO Telehealth (2006) *Telehealth Survey 2005/2006: Health Staff in the Sioux Lookout Zone Identify their Educational Needs*. Keewaytinook Okimakanak, KO Telehealth.

Koelen, M. A. and Lindstrom, B. (2005) Making healthy choices easy choices: The role of empowerment. *Nutrition and Dietetics* 59 (Suppl. 1): S10–16.

Kongshem, L. (1998) Censorware: How well does internet filtering software protect students? *In Electronic School Online*. Available online: http://www.electronic-school.com/0198f1.html (accessed 27 August 2007).

Kouame, G., Harris, M. and Murray, S. (2005) Consumer health information from both sides of the reference desk. *Library Trends* 53: 464–79.

Kovacs, D. K. (2004) Why develop web-based health information workshops for consumers? *Library Trends* 53: 348–59.

Krumholz, H. M., Currie, P. M., Riegel, B., Phillips, C., Petersen, E., Smith, R., Yancy, C. and Faxon, D. (2006) A taxonomy for disease management: A scientific statement from the American Heart Association Disease Management Taxonomy Writing Group. *Circulation* 114: 1432–45.

Lash, S. (2002) *Critique of Information*. London, Sage.

Latour, B. (2005) *Reassembling the Social: An Introduction to Actor-Network-Theory*. Oxford, Oxford University Press.

Lawton, S., Roberts, A. and Gibb, C. (2005) Supporting the parents of children with atopic eczema. *British Journal of Nursing* 14:13: 693.

Leape, L. L. and Berwick, D. M. (2005) Five years after to err is human. *Journal of the American Medical Association* 293(14): 2384–90.

Leydon, G. M., Boulton, M., Moynihan, C., Jones, A., Mossman, J., Boudioni and McPherson, K. (2000) Cancer patients' information needs and information seeking behaviour: In-depth interview study. *British Medical Journal* 320(7239): 909–13.

Lin, J. C. (1999) Applying telecommunication technology to health-care delivery. *Engineering in Medicine and Biology Magazine, IEEE* 18: 28–31.

Livingstone, S. (2003) *The Changing Nature and Uses of Media Literacy, MEDIA@LSE Electronic Working Papers 4*. London, London School of Economics and Political Science.

Lorig, K., Sobel, D. S., Stewart, A. L., Brown Jr., B. W., Bandura, A., Ritter, P., Gonzalez, V. M., Laurent, D. D. and Holman, H. R. (1999) Evidence suggesting that a chronic disease self-management program can improve health status while reducing hospitalization: A randomized trial. *Medical Care* 37: 5–14.

Lupton, D. (1994) Consumerism, commodity culture and health promotion. *Health Promotion International* 9(2): 111–18.

Lussier, M. and Richard, C. (2004) Doctor–patient communication: Getting started. *Canadian Family Physician* 50(3): 361–3.

MacDonald, D., Priddle, M. and Neville, D. (2005) Community pharmacists' expectations of a pharmacy network A baseline evaluation. *Canadian Pharmacists Journal* 138(5): 50.

Maclean, H. (1994) Coming full circle: Home economics and health promotion. Beth Empry Lecture. Edmonton, Alberta, October.

MacLean, R. and Russell, A. (2005) Innovative ways of responding to the information needs of people with MS. *British Journal of Nursing* 14(14): 754–7.

Manchester City Council (2006) *Conditions of Computer Use*. Available online: http://www.manchester.gov.uk/Libraries/usingthelibrary/ict/conditions.htm (accessed 27 August 2007).

Mandl, K. D., Szolovits, P. and Kohane, I. S. (2001) Public standards and patients' control: How to keep electronic medical records accessible but private. *British Medical Journal* 322: 283–7.

Martin, S. (2004) Two thirds of physicians use web in clinical practice. *Canadian Medical Association Journal* 170(1): 28.

Masi, C. M., Suarez-Balcazar, Y., Cassey, M. Z., Kinney, L. and Piotrowski, Z. H. (2003) Internet access and empowerment. A community-based health initiative. *Journal of General Internal Medicine* 18(7): 525–30.

McCulla, K. (2004) *A Comparative Review of Community Health Representatives: Scope of Practice in International Indigenous Communities*. Kahnawake, QC, NIICHRO. Available online: http://www.niichro.com/2004/pdf/international-chr-study.pdf (accessed 1 January 2007).

McFarlane, M., Salyers Bull, S. and Rietmeijer, C. A. (2000) The Internet as a newly emerging risk environment for sexually transmitted diseases. *Journal of the American Medical Association* 284: 443–6.

McFarlane, M., Salyers Bull, S. and Rietmeijer, C. A. (2002) Young adults on the Internet: Risk behaviors for sexually transmitted diseases and HIV. *Journal of Adolescent Health* 31(1): 11–16.

McKeown, L. (2006) *The Daily*. Ottawa, Statistics Canada. Available online: http://www.statcan.ca/Daily/English/060815/d060815b.htm (accessed August 2007).

McLeod, S. D. (1998) The quality of medical information on the Internet: A new public health concern. *Archives of Ophthalmology*, 116(12).

Meeks, B. N. and McCullagh, D. B. (1996) Keys to the kingdom. *Cyberwire Dispatch*. Available online: http://cyberwerks.com/cyberwire/cwd/cwd.96.07.03.html (accessed 27 August 2007).

Miles, A., Loughlin, M. and Polychronis, M. B. (2007) Medicine and evidence: Knowledge and action in clinical practice. *Journal of Evaluation in Clinical Practice* 13: 481–503.

Mimiaga, M. J., Tetu, A., Novak, D., Adelson, S., Vanderwarker, R. and Mayer, K. H. (2006) Acceptability and utility of a partner notification system for sexually transmitted infection exposure using an Internet-based, partner-seeking website for men who have sex with men. *Sixteenth International AIDS Conference*. Toronto, Ontario.

Moore, A., Allen, B., Campbell, S. C. and Carlson, R. A. (2005) Report of the ACR task force on international teleradiology. *Journal of the American College of Radiologists* 2: 121–5.

Morrison, J. (1986) *Treaty Research Report, Treaty No. 9 (1905–1906)*. Treaties and Historical Research Centre, Indian and Northern Affairs Canada.

Moser, I. and Law, J. (2006) Fluids or flows? Information and qualculation in medical practice. *Information Technology & People* 19: 55–73.

Mul, J. de (1999) The informatization of the worldview. *Information, Communication & Society* 2(1): 69–94.

Muller, H.-M., Kenney, E. E. and Sternberg, P. W. (2004) Textpresso: An ontology-based information retrieval and extraction system for biological literature. *PLoS Biology* 2(11): 1984–98.

Murray, S. J., Holmes, D., Perron, A. and Rail, G. (2007) No exit? Intellectual integrity under the regime of 'evidence' and 'best-practices'. *Journal of Evaluation in Clinical Practice* 13: 512–16.

Mykhalovskiy, E., McCoy, L. and Bresalier, M. (2004) Compliance/adherence, HIV, and the critique of medical power. *Social Theory & Health* 2(4): 315–40.

National Aboriginal and Torres Strait Islander Health Council (2003) *National Strategic Framework for Aboriginal and Torres Strait Islander Health: Framework for Action by Governments*. Canberra, National Aboriginal and Torres Strait Islander Health Council.

National Health Information Management Advisory Council (2001) *Health Online: A Health Information Action Plan for Australia*. Canberra, Department of Health and Aged Care.

National Health Strategy Working Party (1989) *National Aboriginal Health Strategy*. Canberra, Office Aboriginal and Torres Strait Islander Health.

National Rural Health Alliance (2006) *Position Paper: Aboriginal and Torres Strait Islander Health Workers*. Canberra, National Rural Health Alliance.

National Rural Health Policy Sub-committee and National Rural Health Alliance (2002) *Healthy Horizons: A Framework for Improving the Health of Rural, Regional and Remote Australians 2003–2007*. Canberra, Australian Health Ministers Conference.

Nettleton, S. and Burrows, R. (2003) E-scaped medicine? Information, reflexivity and health. *Critical Social Policy* 23(2): 165–85.

Nettleton, S. Burrows, R. and O'Malley, L. (2005) The mundane realities of the everyday lay use of the internet for health, and their consequences for media convergence. *Sociology of Health & Illness* 27(7): 972–92.

Nettleton, S., Burrows, R., O'Malley, L. and Watt, I. (2004) Health e-types? An analysis of the everyday use of the internet for health. *Information, Communication & Society* 7: 531–53.

Norfolk, A. (2007) Obese boy is allowed to stay with his mother. *The Times* (London), 28 February, Home News, 11.

Nova Scotia College of Pharmacists. (2007) Code of Ethics. Available online: http://www.nspharmacists.ca/ethics/index.html (accessed 26 July 2007).

Novak, D. S. (2004) *Report: Massachusetts and Manhunt.net partnership*. The Commonwealth of Massachusetts, Department of Public Health, Division of STD Prevention.

O'Kane, M. E. (2002) A strong dose of information: Health plans as 'infomediaries'. *Managed Care Quarterly* 10(2): 1–2.

OFCOM (2005) *Media Literacy Bulletin* 3. London, OFCOM.

Paavolaa, S., Hakkarainen, K. and Sintonen, M. (2006) Abduction with dialogical and trialogical means. *Logic Journal of the IGPL* 14:137–50.

Palella, F. J., Baker, R. K, Moorman, A. C., Chmiel, J. S., Wood, K. C., Brooks, J. T. and Holmberg, S. D. for the HIV Outpatient Study Investigators (2006) Mortality in the highly active antiretroviral therapy era: changing causes of death and disease in the HIV Outpatient Study. *Journal of Acquired Immune Deficiency Syndromes* 43(1): 27–34.

Palella, F. J., Delaney, K., Moorman, A., Loveless, M. O., Fuhrer, J., Satten, G. A., Aschman, D. J. and Holmberg, S. D., for the HIV Outpatient Study Investigators (1998) Declining morbidity and mortality among patients with advanced human immunodeficiency virus infection. *New England Journal of Medicine* 338(13): 853–60.

Pash, R. (2006) Free filters, cash to halt porn tide. *Australian IT*, 21 June. Available online: http://australianit.news.com.au/articles/0,7204,19542040%5E16123%5E%5Enbv%5E,00.html (accessed 27 August 2007).

Patelis, K. (2000) E-mediation by America Online, *in* R. Rogers (ed.) *Preferred Placement*. Maastricht, Jan van Eyck Akademie, 49–63.

Peterson, A. and Lupton, D. (1996) *The New Public Health: Health and Self in the Age of Risk*. London, Sage.

Pew Internet and Family Life Project (2005) *Health Information Online*. Washington, DC, Pew Foundation.

Pezzin, P. L. E., McDonald, M. V., Peng, T., Feldman, H. and Murtaugh, C. M. (2005) Just-in-time. Evidence-based e-mail reminders in home health care: Impact on patient outcomes. *Health Services Research* 40(3): 865–85.

Pitts, V. (2004) Illness and internet empowerment: Writing and reading breast cancer in cyberspace. *Health* 8(1): 33–59.

Pong, R. W., Saunders, D., Church, J., Wanke, M. and Cappon, P. (1995) *Health Human Resources in Community-Based Health Care: A Review of the Literature*. Ottawa, Health Canada. Available online: http://hc-sc.gc.ca/hcs-sss/pubs/care-soins/1995-build-plan-commun/build-plan-commun1/index_e.html (accessed 1 January 2007).

Productivity Commission (2005) *Australia's Health Workforce*. Canberra, Research Report.

Prosser, B. (2006) Summary of Preliminary Findings from the Third Omnibus Survey – October, 2005 to November, 2005. Unpublished internal report, QUILTS.

Public Health Agency of Canada (2006) *HIV and AIDS in Canada: Surveillance Report to December 31, 2005* [April]. Available online: http://www.phac-aspc.gc.ca/publicat/aids-sida/haic-vsac1205/index.html (accessed 11 October 2006).

Public Health Information Development Unit (2001)*ASGC Remoteness Classification, Australia*. Adelaide, Public Health Information Development Unit.

Queensland Health (1994) *Aboriginal and Torres Strait Islander Health Policy*. Brisbane, Queensland Health.

Queensland Health (1999) *Queensland Health Indigenous Workforce Management Strategy*. Brisbane, Queensland Health.

Ramirez, R., Aitkin, H., Jamieson, R. and Richardson, D. (2003) *Harnessing ICTS: A Canadian First Nations Experience – Introduction to K-Net*. Institute for Connectivity in the Americas, Ottawa, IDRC. Available online: http://www.eldis.org/static/DOC15297.htm (accessed 1 January 2007).

RAND Health (2001) *Proceed With Caution: A Report on the Quality of Health Information on the Internet: Complete Study*. Oakland, CA, California Health Care Foundation. Available online: http://www.chcf.org/documents/consumer/Proceed WithCautionCompleteStudy.pdf (accessed 22 October 2007).

Ratib, O., Swiernik, M. and McCoy, J. M. (2003) From PACS to integrated EMR. *Computerized Medical Imaging and Graphics* 27: 207–15.

Reif, S. Golin, C. E. and Smith, S. R. (2005) Barriers to accessing HIV/AIDS care in North Carolina: Rural and urban differences. *AIDS Care* 17(5): 558–65.

Report on the First Nations Telehealth Workshop (2002) *Building a Telehealth Toolkit for Sioux Lookout Zone Communities*. Sioux Lookout, ON, 22–23 October.

Rhodes, S. D. (2004) Hookups or health promotion? An exploratory study of a chat room-based HIV prevention intervention for men who have sex with men. *AIDS Education and Prevention* 16(4): 315–27.

Rhodes, S. D., Hergenrather, K. C., Ramsey, B., Yee, L. and Wilkin, A. (2006) The development of a cyber-based education and referral/men for men (cyber/M4M): A chat room-based intervention to prevent HIV infection among gay men and MSM. *Sixteenth International AIDS Conference*, Toronto, Ontario.

Rideout, V. (2001) *Kaiser Family Foundation Survey: Generation Rx: How Young People Use the Internet for Health Information* [electronic version]. California, Kaiser Family Foundation.

Rideout, V. (2005) *E-health and the Elderly: How Seniors Use the Internet for Health Information* [electronic version]. Washington, DC, Kaiser Family Foundation.

Rideout, V., Richardson, C. and Resnick, P. (2002) *See-No-Evil: How Internet Filters Affect the Search for Online Health Information* (Executive Summary) [electronic version]. Washington, DC, Kaiser Family Foundation.

Rose, J. and Jones, M. (2005) The double dance of agency: A socio-theoretic account of how machines and humans interact. *Systems, Signs & Actions* 1: 27–43.

Ross, C. S. and Nilsen, K. (2000) Has the internet changed anything in reference? *Reference & User Services Quarterly* 40: 147–55.

Ross, J. W. (1995) Hospital social work, *in* R. L. Edwards (ed.), *Encyclopedia of Social Work*. Washington, NASW. 1365–77.

Rowlandson, J. (2005) *Position Paper: Turning the Corner with First Nations Tele-health*. Keewaytinook Okimakanak. Available online: http://telehealth.knet.ca/modules/ContentExpress/img_repository/KOTelehealth_Position_Paper_6May.pdf (accessed 1 January 2007).

Royal Pharmaceutical Society of Great Britain (2004) Press release. *Code of Ethics Updated to Reflect CPD and Online Pharmacy Requirements*. Available online: http://www.rpsgb.org/pdfs/pr041214.pdf (accessed 13 August 2007).

Salyers Bull, S., McFarlane, M. and King, D. (2001) Barriers to STD/HIV prevention on the Internet. *Health Education Research* 16(6): 661–70.

Savage, A. L. and Auld, G. W. (2006) Development and evaluation of education materials promoting local Colorado foods. *Journal of Nutrition Education and Behaviour* 38: 61–2.

Schanzer, D. L. (2003) Trends in HIV/AIDS mortality in Canada. *Canadian Journal of Public Health* 94(2): 135–9.

Seaby, C. (2002) *Aboriginal Health Care in Northern Ontario: The Role of the Nurse in the Transferred Communities 1986–2001*. Ottawa, University of Ottawa. Available online: http://www.med.uottawa.ca/medweb/hetenyi/seaby.htm (accessed 1 January 2007).

Selwyn, N. (2003) Apart from technology: Understanding people's non-use of information and communication technologies in everyday life. *Technology in Society* 25: 99–116.

Semchuk, W. (2004) Empowering providers to meet patient information needs: Reduce patient anxiety to support adherence. *Canadian Pharmacists Journal* 137(3): 46.

Shulman, L. (2000) Beginning and the contracting skills, *in* N. E. Sullivan, K. Steinhouse and B. Gelfand, (eds.) *Challenges for Social Work Students: Skills, Knowledge and Values*, Toronto, Canadian Scholars Press, pp. 127–44.

Sidorov, J. (2006) It ain't necessarily so: The electronic health record and the unlikely prospect of reducing health care costs. *Health Affairs* 25: 1079–85.

Silverman, J., Kurtz, S. M. and Draper, J. (2005) *Skills for Communicating with Patients*. Oxford, Radcliffe.

Silverstone, R. (1999) *Why Study the Media?* London, Sage.

Skinner, H., Biscope, S. and Poland, B. (2003) Quality of Internet access: Barrier behind Internet use statistics. *Social Science & Medicine* 57(5): 875–80.

Social Health Reference Group (2004) *Social and Emotional Well-being Frame-work: A National Strategic Framework for Aboriginal and Torres Strait Islander Peoples' Mental Health and Social and Emotional Well-being 2004–2009*. Canberra, National Aboriginal and Torres Strait Islander Health Council and National Mental Health Working Group.

Sommerland, E., Child, C., Ramsden, C. and Kelleher, J. (2004) *An Evaluation of the People's Network and ICT Training for Public Library Staff Programme. Books and Bytes: New Service Paradigms for the 21st Century Library*. London, Tavistock Institute.

Song, J. and Zahedi, F. M. (2007) Trust in health infomediaries. *Decision Support Systems* 43: 390–407.

Standing Committee on Aboriginal and Torres Strait Islander Health (2002) *Aboriginal and Torres Strait Islander Health Workforce National Strategic Framework*. Canberra, Aboriginal Health Ministers' Advisory Council.

Star, S. L. (1995) Introduction, *in* S. L. Star (ed.) *The Cultures of Computing*. Oxford, Blackwell, pp. 1–28.

Stark, P. B. (2006) Expert Report of Phillip B. Stark, PhD, *in ACLU v. Gonzales* (Civ. Action No. 98–5591 (E.D. Pa.)) 8 May 2006. Available online: http://sethf.com/infothought/blog/archives/copa-censorware-stark-report.pdf (accessed 27 August 2007).

State Library of Queensland (2006) *Internet Public Use Policy*. Available online: http://www.slq.qld.gov.au/about/pub/pol (accessed 27 August 2007).

State Library of Western Australia (2005) *Public Internet Access Policy*. Available online: http://www.liswa.wa.gov.au/pdf/publicinternetpolicymar05.pdf (accessed 27 August 2007).

Statistics Canada (2005) *Household Internet Use, by Location of Access, by Province: British Columbia*. CANSIM, table 358–0002. Ottawa, Statistics Canada. Available online: http://www40.statcan.ca/l01/cst01/comm12k.htm (accessed 17 June 2006).

Stedman's Medical Dictionary for the Health Professions and Nursing, 5th Ed. (2005) Philadelphia, Lippincott Williams & Wilkins.

Stewart, J. (2007) Local experts in the domestication of information and communication technologies. *Information, Communication & Society* 10(4): 547–69.

Struthers, R. (2000) The lived experience of Ojibwa and Cree women healers. *Journal of Holistic Nursing* 18(3): 261–79.

Su, K. C., Waldron, S. E. and Patrick, T. B. (2004) Differences in the effects of filters on health information retrieval from the Internet in three languages from three countries: A comparative study. *Medinfo* 11(Part II): 1313–17.

Sullivan, D. (2006) *comScore Media Metrix Search Engine Ratings*. Available online: http://searchenginewatch.com/showPage.html?page=2156431 (accessed 24 July 2006).

Sutherland, J. and Gibson, E. (in press) Guiding patrons to online health information: Can librarians be found liable? *Canadian Journal of Library and Information Sciences*.

Tan, H. and Ng, J. H. K. (2006) Googling for diagnosis. *British Medical Journal* 333: 1143–5.

Thompson, J. B. (1995) *The Media and Modernity*. Stanford, CA, Stanford University Press.

Tikkanen, R. and Ross, M. W. (2003) Technological tearoom trade: Characteristics of Swedish men visiting gay Internet chat rooms. *AIDS Education and Prevention* 15(2): 122–32.

Tregenza, J. and Abbott, K. (1995) *Rhetoric and Reality: Perceptions of the Roles of AHWs in Central Australia*. Alice Springs, NT, Central Australian Aboriginal Congress.

Trudgen, R. (2000) *Why Warriors Lie Down and Die: Towards an Understanding of Why the Aboriginal People of Arnhem Land Face the Greatest Crisis in Health and Education Since European Contact*. Parap, NT, Aboriginal Resource and Development Services Inc.

United Kingdom Library Association (1998) *Access to Information: Freedom and Censorship*. Available online: http://www.la-hq.org.uk/directory/prof_issues/ifac.html (accessed 27 August 2007).

United Kingdom Library Association (2000) *Guidance Notes on the Use of Filtering Software in Libraries.* Available online: http://www.la-hq.org.uk/directory/prof_issues/filter2.html (accessed 27 August 2007).

United States Equal Employment Opportunity Commission (2007) *Harassment.* Available online: http://www.eeoc.gov/types/harassment.html (accessed 27 August 2007).

United States v. American Library Association, 114 Stat. 2763A–335 (2000).

United States v. American Library Association, 123 S. Ct. 2297 (2003).

Veenhof, B., Clermont, Y. and Sciadas, G. (2005) *Literacy and Digital Technologies: Linkages and Outcomes.* Ottawa, Statistics Canada. Available online: http://www.statcan.ca/english/research/56F0004MIE/56F0004MIE2005012.pdf (accessed 27 July 2006).

Verheijden, M. W., Bakx, J. C., Van Weel, C. and Van Staveren, W. A. (2005) Potentials and pitfalls for nutrition counseling in general practice. *European Journal of Clinical Nutrition* 59: S122–9.

Wahab, S. (2005) Motivational interviewing and social work practice. *Journal of Social Work* 5:1 45–60.

Wald, H. S., Dube, C. E. and Anthony, D. C. (2007) Untangling the Web: The impact of Internet use on health care and the physician–patient relationship. *Patient Education and Counseling* 68(3): 218–24.

Wathen, C. N. (2006a) Alternatives to hormone replacement therapy: A multimethod study of women's experiences. *Complementary Therapies in Medicine* 14(3): 185–92.

Wathen, C. N. (2006b) Health information seeking in context: How women make decisions regarding hormone replacement therapy. *Journal of Health Communication* 11: 477–93.

Wathen, C. N. and Burkell, J. (2002) Believe it or not: Factors influencing credibility on the Web. *Journal of the American Society for Information Science and Technology* 53(2): 134–44.

Wathen, C. N. and Harris, R. M. (2007) 'I try to take care of it myself.' How rural women search for health information. *Qualitative Health Research* 17(5): 639–51.

Weiner, S. J., Barnet, B., Cheng, T. L. and Daaleman, T. P. (2005) Processes for effective communication in primary care. *Annals of Internal Medicine* 142: 709–14.

Weinstein, M. D., Descour, M. R., Liang, C., Bhattacharyya, A. K., Graham, A. R., Davis, J. R., Scott, K. M., Richter, L., Krupinski, E. A., Szymus, J., Kayser, K. and Dunn, B. E. (2001) Telepathology overview: From concept to implementation. *Human Pathology* 32: 1283–99.

Wessel, J., Balint, J., Crill, C. and Klotz, K. (2005) Standards for specialized nutrition support: hospitalized pediatric patients. *Nutrition in Clinical Practice* 20(1): 103–16.

West, D. S., Herbert, D. A. and Knowlton, C. H. (2000) The practice of community pharmacy, *in* A. R. Gennaro et al. (eds) *Remington: The Science and Practice of Pharmacy.* Philadelphia, Lipincott, Williams and Wilkins, pp. 28–32.

William, W., Simons, W. W., Mandl, K. D. and Kohane, I. S. (2005) The PING personally controlled electronic medical record system: Technical architecture. *Journal of the American Medical Informatics Association* 12(1): 47–54.

Williams, R. (1977) *Marxism and Literature.* Oxford, Oxford University Press.

Williamson, K. (1998) Discovered by chance: The role of incidental information acquisition in an ecological model of information use. *Library and Information Science Research* 20(1): 23–40.

Wilson, K. (2001) Therapeutic landscapes and First Nations Peoples: An exploration of culture, health and place. *Health and Place* 9: 83–93.

Winkler, M. F. (2005) Improving safety and reducing harm associated with specialized nutrition support. *Nutrition in Clinical Practice* 20: 595–6.

Winter, M. (1988) *The Culture and Control of Expertise: Toward a Sociological Understanding of Librarianship*. New York, Greenwood Press.

Woolf, S. H. and Johnson, R. E. (2005) The break-even point: When medical advances are less important than improving the fidelity with which they are delivered. *Annals of Family Medicine* 3(6): 545–52.

Wyatt, S. and Henwood, F. (2006) 'The best bones in the graveyard': Risky technologies and risks in knowledge, *in* C. Timmerman and J. Anderson (eds) *Devices & Designs: Medical Innovation in Historical Perspective*. Basingstoke, Palgrave Macmillan, pp. 231–48.

Wyatt, S., Henwood, F., Hart, A. and Smith, J. (2005) The digital divide, health information and everyday life. *New Media and Society* 7(2): 199–218.

Wyatt, S., Thomas, G. and Terranova, T. (2002) They came, they surfed, they went back to the beach: Conceptualizing use and non-use of the internet, *in* S. Woolgar (ed.) *Virtual Society? Technology, Cyberpole, Reality*. Oxford, Oxford University Press, pp. 23–40.

Zhang, J., Sun, J., Yang, Y., Chen, X., Meng, L. and Lian P. (2005) Web-based electronic patient records for collaborative medical applications. *Comparative Medical Imaging and Graphics* 29: 115–24.

Index

213

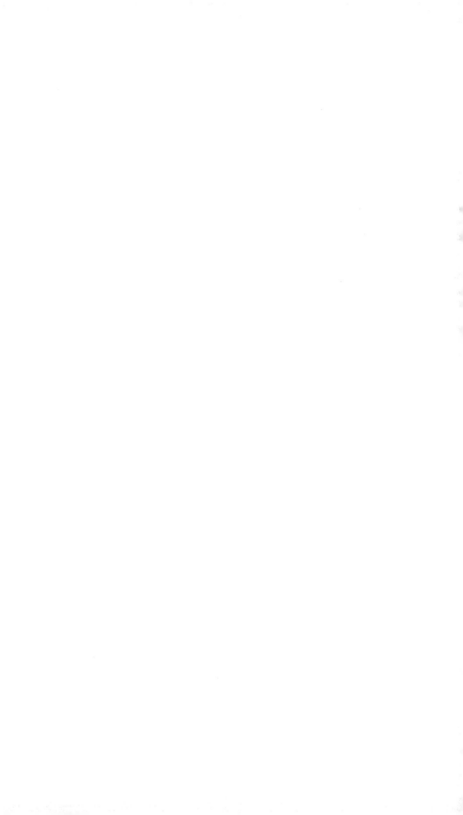